LEAN IN 15

JOE WICKS

The Body Coach

First published 2015 by Bluebird
an imprint of Pan Macmillan
20 New Wharf Road, London N1 9RR
Associated companies throughout the world
www.panmacmillan.com

ISBN 978-1-5098-0066-7

Grateful acknowledgement is made to 'My Lean Winners' and the 'Lean in 15 Heroes' for permission to include the images on pages 207–11, 216–17 and 222–3.

2 2

A CIP catalogue record for this book is available from the British Library.

Printed in Italy

Designed and Typeset by www.cabinlondon.co.uk

CONTENTS

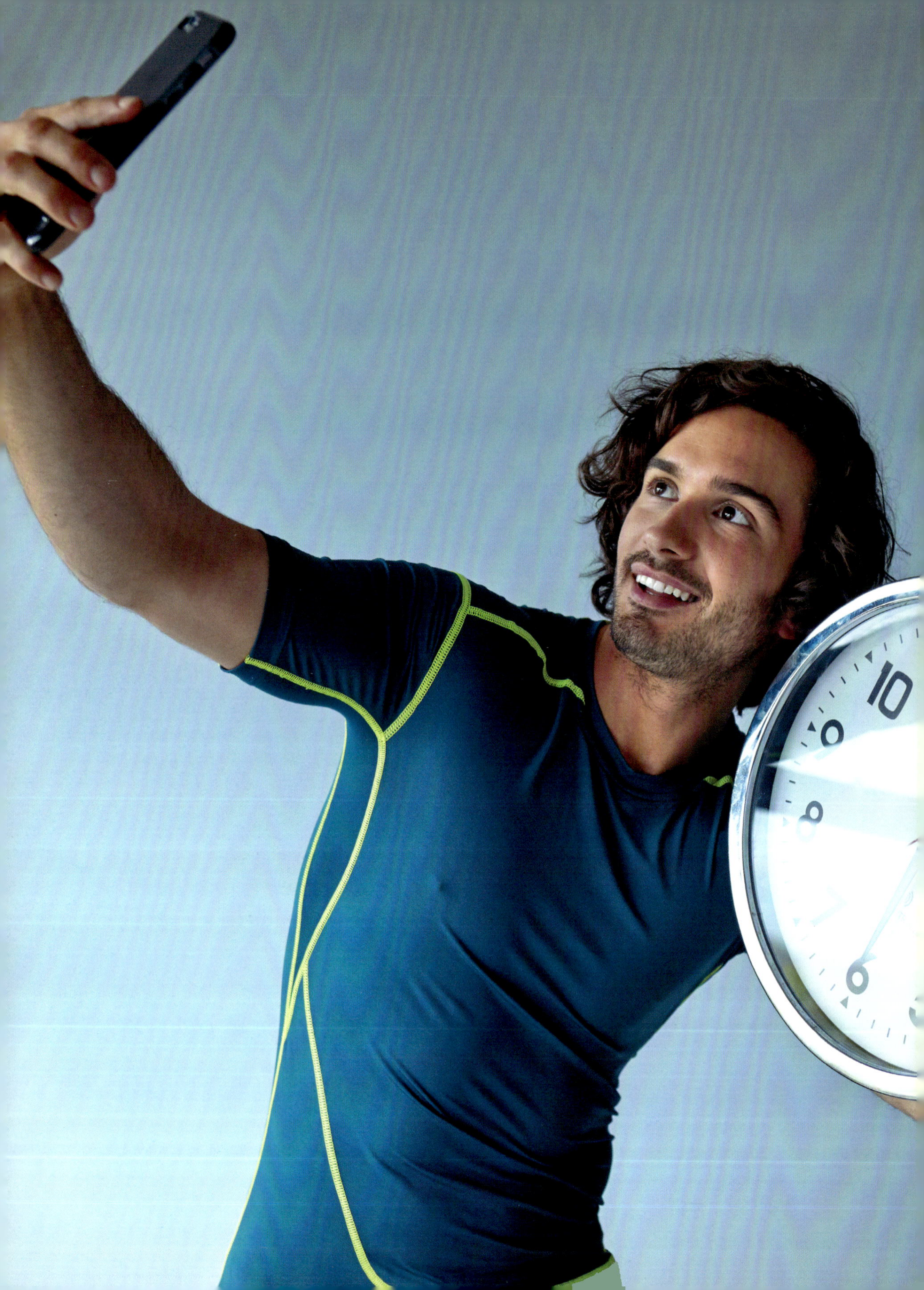

A LITTLE BIT ABOUT ME

When I posted my first ever #Leanin15 video on Instagram in early 2014, I never imagined it would lead to me writing this book. It all started as a bit of fun in my kitchen, with the idea of sharing simple recipes to help people get lean.

> ‘I saw every meal as an opportunity to share a new recipe’

All of the meals were ready in 15 minutes, and the videos were only 15 seconds long . . . hence the hashtag #Leanin15. To begin with, no one was watching my videos, and my neighbours thought I was mad. They often heard me singing or shouting, ‘Bosh, that's Lean in 15’ and ‘Oooh, midget trees’ (that's what I call broccoli, by the way!).

Some of my friends thought it was stupid, and said I should get back to doing personal training and running my boot camps – that's what I had been happily doing for the past 5 years. But I was having fun, so I just carried on anyway, often posting up to 3 videos a day. It took a lot of time and energy to stop and film everything I cooked, but I saw every meal as an opportunity to share a new recipe, and this was my motivation to keep going.

To my surprise, within a few months, hundreds of thousands of people all over the world were following along, making my recipes at home and sharing them online. I think the speed and simplicity of my meals, along with the fact that I was clearly enjoying myself, inspired so many people to get involved.

I'm completely self-taught when it comes to cooking, so I never over-complicate things. I use foods that anyone can find in their local supermarket and this makes Lean in 15 accessible to everyone and perfect for busy people.

My approach is also about making small lifestyle changes rather than following a strict regime. I often post photos of myself eating out in restaurants and enjoying treats. I do love a chocolate fondant – guilty as charged!

I think people respond well to me, because I don't eat perfectly all the time, and I never pretend that I do. In fact, my diet used to be pretty shocking. I've always trained hard, but I didn't really take my nutrition seriously. Like most busy people, I was lazy when it came to cooking and used lack of time as an excuse. I often ate cereal, sandwiches on the go and ready meals. This left me feeling tired, but I just accepted it as normal. I drank fizzy drinks and snacked on chocolate bars in between personal training clients. During this time, my body didn't change much and I could never get lean. Eventually, I discovered that no matter how hard I trained, I couldn't out-train a poor diet.

'My approach is also about making small lifestyle changes rather than a strict regime'

It was only when I really started to study nutrition after university that I realized just how important real food was for my energy levels and making changes in my body. The more I understood, the more I started to transform my own body. With this new knowledge and understanding of nutrition, I was able to get lean and stay lean. I then started to apply my knowledge with my clients, and it was remarkable how quickly their bodies would respond. Helping clients get fast transformations meant I soon got fully booked as a personal trainer. But, even with two busy boot camps, I could only ever work with about 100 people each week. This wasn't enough for me. I wanted to help more people reach their goals, so I started putting more energy into my social media. With Twitter, Facebook, YouTube and Instagram, I was able to reach thousands of people at once by sharing content online – video recipes, workouts and blogs. As my social media following grew, I started to realize just how shocking the diet industry really was. Every day I would receive messages from people on all sorts of depressing low-calorie crash diets, and it soon became apparent just how much wrong information people were being given – and how far they were willing to go to lose weight. Regimes of training for 2 hours a day and eating fewer than 1000 kcal were way too common, and it upset me that people were living this way, always trying to find a shortcut and never getting the results they wanted. Very unhappy people were being held prisoner to diets that would never give them the lean body they wanted. I believe such crash diets are a contributory factor to so many of the eating disorders and body image issues we face today. People have become convinced that the only way to lose body fat is to drastically cut calories to create a huge energy deficit – but this only leads to yo-yo dieting and people battling their weight for years, which is not a healthy way to live, and it shouldn't be accepted as the norm.

> 'MY AIM WAS TO CREATE A SUSTAINABLE PLAN'

One day while I was out jogging, I decided I would do something about it. I would create an online nutrition and training plan to educate people properly and rescue them from these damaging, unhealthy diets. My aim was to create a sustainable plan with tasty meals that would get people eating more food, training more effectively (and for much less time!) and burning fat.

Everyone has different energy demands. My meal plans are unique; I create tailored meal plans that allow choice and flexibility, to ensure people get results and keep them. After months of planning, the 90 Day Shift, Shape and Sustain plan was born. I used social media to promote it, and started to post 'before' and 'after' transformation pictures, along with written testimonials. I had no idea what I had created at the time – and, to this day, I can't quite believe the success it's had. But by creating an online community, I unknowingly connected thousands of people who were all on the same journey. As more and more clients signed up online, I had to step away from my boot camps, and eventually I passed on all my personal training clients to a friend. My business was now fully online and going global.

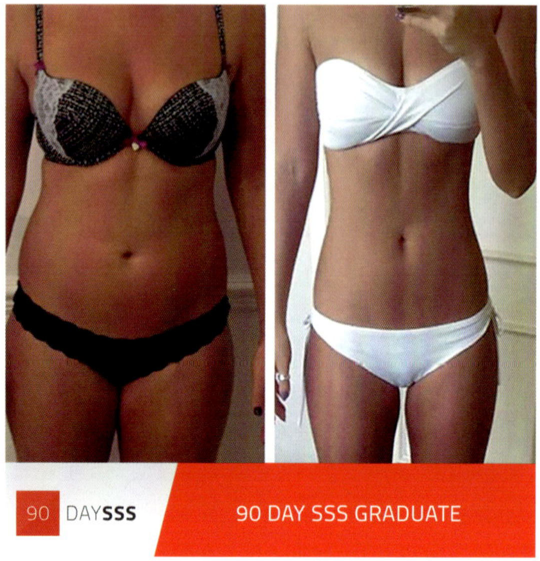

Originally it was mainly people from the UK signing up, but then people all over the world started to get on board. Places as far away as Australia, Sweden, Singapore and Dubai were starting to hear about Lean in 15 and signing up to my 90 Day Shift, Shape and Sustain plan. It started off with just me answering a few emails and sending a few plans out each week, but before I knew it I had thousands of people signing up each month and a team of support staff to help coach clients on their journey.

I absolutely love what I do now, and although I never get to actually meet any of my clients, I'm really proud of all of them and feel inspired by them every day. By educating people on nutrition I have been able to empower them to take control and achieve their goals in a healthy and enjoyable way.

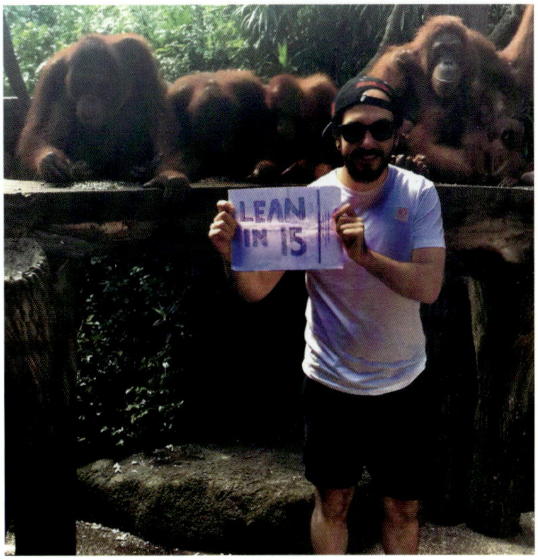

> I am now on a mission to help even more people

As The Body Coach, I am now on a mission to help even more people. It's important to note that my online business didn't just happen overnight – it grew organically and came from nothing but hard work. It takes a lot of trust for a person to buy into something without ever meeting you, and I built that trust up over hundreds of hours of interaction, videos and tweets. When no one was listening, I kept sharing and giving, and eventually people started to hear me.

So that's a little bit about me and my story up to now. I'm very excited to be sharing my knowledge and recipes with you. I hope you enjoy the book and get inspired to cook, prep like a boss and get the body you've always wanted.

Joe Wicks

- THE BODY COACH

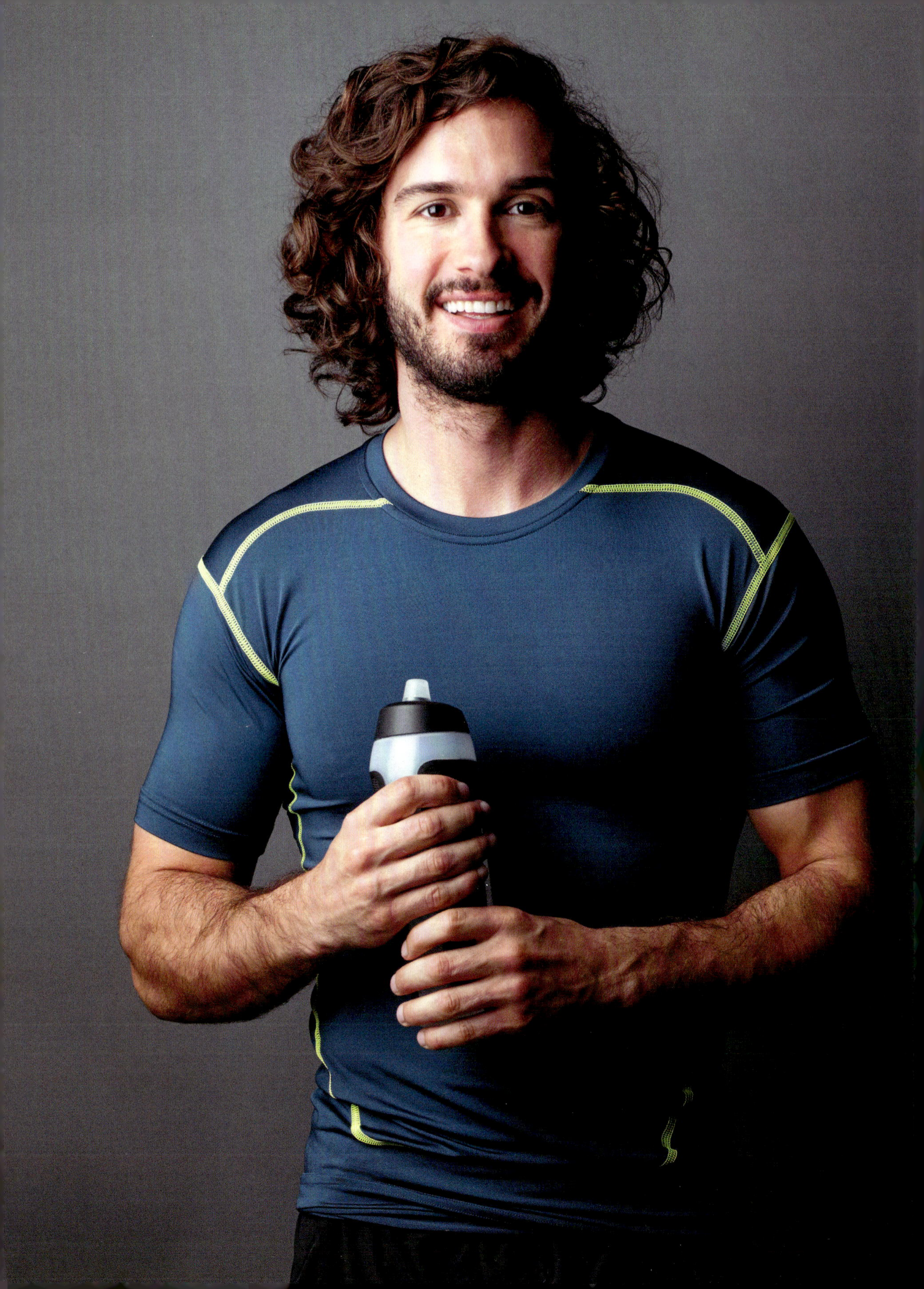

1

THE LEAN IN 15 PLAN

DIETS DON'T WORK!

> Success only happens when a programme is enjoyable and sustainable

The problem with diets is that they don't work – not in the long term, anyway. Yes, you can lose weight initially, especially with a drastic decrease in calories, but the likelihood is that you will soon return to your old eating habits and regain any weight lost. After working with thousands of clients, I know that success only happens when a programme is enjoyable and sustainable. A meal plan needs to be easy to follow and stress-free, because life is stressful enough and we simply don't have the time to spend hours in the kitchen every day.

This is why I created Lean in 15. No matter how busy you are, you can take control and find a quarter of an hour to cook your meals and stay lean. This isn't a strict diet – it's a lifestyle that will transform your body and the way you eat forever. Once I teach you how to fuel your body properly, you will never need to follow a low-calorie diet again.

Most of the recipes in this book will be ready in less than 15 minutes, and many of them can be batch-cooked, so you can double up and prepare meals for the day or week ahead. A few of the meals take a little longer than 15 minutes so are not technically 'Lean in 15' but don't worry, it's because they taste great and will be well worth the wait! The busier you are, the more you will need to prep your meals. I call this 'Prepping like a boss', and it's one of the ways you can guarantee your success. I'll be sharing my top tips for prepping like a boss further on in this book, so keep a lookout.

There are no shortcuts

I want you to ignore all the adverts trying to sell you fat-burning herbal supplements, meal-replacement shakes or juice diets. They are not the solution. In fact, these diets are the problem, as they go against the basic principles of nutrition and the way metabolism works. What's more, they rely on repeat business, because they know that once you lose the weight, you'll soon regain it and be back for more of their products. I want to help you break this vicious circle once and for all.

> 'I want you to eat *more* food, and I'm going to show you how to fuel your body properly'

The truth is there are no shortcuts to a lean body. It takes time, dedication, consistent training and the right nutrition. The good news is that Lean in 15 is not going to deprive you of entire food groups or leave you feeling hungry like most diets. My approach is the complete opposite. I want to encourage you to think differently and change your approach. I want you to eat *more* food, and I'm going to show you how to fuel your body properly, so you burn fat and build lean muscle. The more lean muscle you have, the more efficient your metabolism will be – and that means you can enjoy eating even more food. That's winning!

I'm also going to explain the importance of fats, proteins and carbohydrates, so you understand what to fuel your body with and when. My philosophy is simple and easy to adopt into your lifestyle.

Your body is unique

The portions in the recipes in this book are not specifically tailored to you, as it would be impossible without knowing much more about you (your current weight, activity level, age range and more). Every body has its own unique energy demands, so you will need to increase or decrease the portion sizes according to your activity levels. For example, if you train hard and have a really physically active job, you need to eat more than someone who sits at a desk for eight hours a day and does little exercise.

> 'Listen to your body – and please don't go hungry'

It doesn't have to be difficult or complicated. You will soon start to notice if you feel energized or not, so listen to your body – and please don't go hungry! Although I can't tailor portion sizes to individual readers, the structured way of eating outlined in this book – what to eat and when – is very effective for fat loss. The structure is the same as cycle one of my 90 Day Shift, Shape and Sustain plan, which has worked brilliantly for tens of thousands of people. This phase is called the 'Shift' phase, because that's exactly what it does. It shifts unwanted fat by putting your body in fat-burning mode at all times through a combination of diet and exercise (I have also included some sample home HIIT workouts for you to try out – see page 194).

Understanding macronutrients

Our three main energy sources – fats, protein and carbohydrates – are called macronutrients. They all play an important role in helping our bodies stay lean, strong and healthy. The way of eating in this book won't cut any of these out of your diet, but rather will provide you with them in the right ratios at the right time to get the best possible response from your body.

During low-intensity activity, such as watching TV, walking to the shops and even sleeping, your body mostly uses fats to fuel itself. When working at a high intensity, it mostly uses stored carbohydrates for energy. I'm going to show you how to use this knowledge to your advantage, to ensure your body is always using the correct energy source in line with your energy demands.

Let's talk about fats

Fats have been unfairly demonized, to the extent that people now believe that all fats are bad and will make you get fat, and a whole industry has arisen around low-fat versions of common foods. Fat is often the first thing people cut out when trying to lose weight. But not all fats are the same. Some fats – such as trans-fats found in processed foods – should be avoided, but others are actually essential for the body, such as omega-3s (found in oily fish), which help reduce inflammation. These are known as essential fatty acids (EFAs), as they cannot be made in the body and so must be obtained from the diet. Fat also plays an essential role in vitamin absorption: vitamins A, D, E and K are fat-soluble, meaning your body can't absorb them without fat being present.

People also often associate energy with carbohydrates, but fats are actually the most energy-dense macronutrient of all. Fats provide your body with 9 kcal energy per gram, compared to just 4 kcal per gram from protein and carbohydrates. This makes fat an incredible energy source, and one that keeps blood sugar levels stable. Fat also takes longer to digest in the body, which means you feel satisfied for longer and are less likely to snack in between meals.

Why are fats important?

Fats have several important roles in the body, including:

- Providing you with energy
- Enabling the absorption of fat-soluble vitamins
- Protecting your organs, nerves and tissues
- Helping to regulate body temperature
- Every cell membrane in the body needs fat for protection, and fat is also needed to grow new healthy cells
- Fats are involved in the production of essential hormones in the body
- Maintenance of healthy hair, skin and nails

What are the types of fat?

There are 3 types of fat:

- Saturated – animal fats, butter, eggs, cheese, coconut oil
- Monounsaturated – nuts, avocados, extra virgin olive oil, peanut oil, sesame oil
- Polyunsaturated – sunflower oil, walnut oil, flaxseed oil, and oily fish such as salmon and mackerel

Saturated fats have an awful reputation, which dates back to the 1950s, when a study found that the consumption of saturated fat increased levels of bad cholesterol in the blood, and that this led to coronary heart disease. In hindsight, this research was extremely flawed and failed to take into account those countries where people had a very high intake of saturated fat and yet very low levels of heart disease. Unfortunately this 'diet-heart' hypothesis influenced government health guidelines and the low-fat food industry started to boom. Instead of fats, we were encouraged to consume more carbohydrates, such as grains, rice and pasta. But since then, deaths from obesity, diabetes and heart-related diseases have continued to rise.

> 'A handful of nuts, seeds or half an avocado make a perfect snack'

Ironically, the latest research suggests that saturated fats from butter, milk, cream, eggs and coconut oil actually increase the levels of good cholesterol in the blood and benefit the heart, so there is no need to fear these foods. This doesn't mean you should sit down and eat a whole wheel of cheese, though. Fats do contain lots of calories, after all, so you need to eat everything in moderation and in line with your own personal energy demands.

Monounsaturated fats

Monounsaturated fats, found in things such as extra virgin olive oil, avocados and nuts, are great for increasing good cholesterol levels. This is one of the reasons a handful of nuts, seeds or half an avocado make a perfect snack. Unlike sugary cereal bars and chocolate, these snacks will also keep your blood sugar levels stable and sustain your energy levels for much longer.

Polyunsaturated fats

Polyunsaturated fats can be found in oily fish like salmon and mackerel and are a great source of omega-3 fatty acids. These are considered anti-inflammatory, which means they reduce your risk of injuries and chronic disease. I'm not the biggest fan of fish, and for the first 25 years of my life I wouldn't go near it, but I've slowly trained myself to eat it because I understand its importance for my health. No amount of omega-3 fish oil capsules will beat a fresh piece of wild salmon, so try to eat fish at least twice a week.

Bad fats

The hydrogenated fats we need to eliminate from our diet aren't just found in sugary sweets, pastries and fast-food restaurants. They are also hidden in many low-fat diet products. Low-fat ready meals, for example, may be low in saturated fat but they are often loaded with hydrogenated trans-fats to increase their shelf-life. My advice is to prepare all of your own meals from scratch, avoiding ready meals wherever possible.

What should I cook with?

You'll notice that I mostly use coconut oil or butter for cooking – this is because these saturated fats are more stable when heated to high temperatures. Processed polyunsaturated vegetable oils and margarines, on the other hand, become unstable when heated. This means they oxidize easily, producing free radicals, and these are not what you want to be putting inside your body. When free radicals attack fat molecules, they develop similar properties to a trans-fat, increasing the levels of bad cholesterol in your blood at the same time as decreasing the levels of good cholesterol – a double-whammy effect that's not great when it comes to the health of your heart.

What about protein?

Protein forms the basis of all meals in the Lean in 15 plan, and remains consistent on both training and rest days. Protein is essential for:

- ★ Maintaining the structure and strength of cells and tissues
- ★ Regulation of metabolism
- ★ Production of hormones
- ★ Repair and growth of muscle tissues
- ★ Strengthening your immune system

> 'Prepare all of your own meals from scratch, avoiding ready meals wherever possible'

Where should I get my protein?

Proteins are broken down into amino acids inside the body. Many of my recipes contain animal protein sources, such as eggs, fish, chicken and beef. These are considered complete protein sources because they contain all the essential amino acids needed by the body. If you are a vegetarian you can of course use tofu or Quorn as a protein source, but you'll need to eat much larger quantities to get your protein intake to the required level.

‘REAL FOOD, NOT DUST, BURNS FAT’

Protein powder

I always say real food, not dust, burns fat. What I mean by this is that supplements should only be used alongside a good diet and not in place of real food. However, you may notice that in some of my recipes, such as overnight oats, I do use protein powder. Whey protein is a brilliant post-workout addition to your diet because it reaches the muscles quickly, so the amino acids can start to repair and rebuild muscle fibres immediately after a training session. If you need a dairy-free alternative (whey is derived from dairy), you could try a vegan protein powder, such as hemp or pea.

Let's talk about carbohydrates

There is so much confusion surrounding carbohydrates – which carbs are good and which are bad, and when you can and can't eat them. I'm going to clear all this up and show you what a great energy source they can be.

We've all heard the ridiculous myth that eating carbs after 6pm makes you fat. It's pure nonsense! Carbs don't make you fat. What actually makes us gain fat is when we eat over and above our bodies' energy demands. So, providing you eat the right amount each day, you will not gain fat but instead will be able to train harder and build more muscle, which will make you leaner.

Why do we need carbohydrates?

- ★ Carbohydrates are the main source of energy for muscles during intense exercise
- ★ They are needed for the proper functioning of the central nervous system, kidneys and muscles
- ★ Carbs also contain fibre, which is important for good intestinal health and digestion
- ★ They are essential for healthy brain function

The white carb police

Lots of people seem to be scared of eating white bread, pasta and rice, and attempt to ban it from their lives. I call these people 'the white carb police'. Unshakeable in their belief that you can't eat white carbs when trying to burn fat, they will eat only the brown, wholegrain versions of these carbs – but you really don't need to fear white carbs.

While it's true that wholegrain carbs have a lower glycaemic load (GL), which means they don't cause your blood sugar levels to spike as much as white carbs, after training your body actually loves high-GL foods. The higher the GL of a food, the greater will be the elevation of blood glucose levels, prompting the pancreas to release insulin. However, this insulin response is great after a workout as it means the nutrients from your carbohydrate-refuel meal are shuttled to the muscles quicker. Combining high GL carbs with low GL carbs such as table sugar with porridge oats reduces the overall GL and elevation of blood sugar levels.

In summary, if you love brown rice, eat brown rice – but if you long for a big bowl of white rice or a white bagel, then know that after you train is the ideal time to enjoy it.

How will I be eating?

You are going to be eating in line with your energy demands. This means that you will eat differently on training days and rest days.

You are going to ensure that your body is using the correct energy source, in line with your energy demands – that is, carbohydrates after exercise, and fats as steady fuel for the remainder of your day and night, and on rest days.

The recipes in this book are broken down into 3 sections:

1. Reduced-carbohydrate meals: rich in healthy fats and protein
2. Post-workout carbohydrate-refuel meals: high in protein and carbohydrates
3. Snacks and treats: sweet and savoury snacks and tasty treats

On a training day, you will eat 2 reduced-carbohydrate meals, 1 post-workout carbohydrate-refuel meal and 2 snacks.

On a rest day, you will eat 3 reduced-carbohydrate meals and 2 snacks.

> 'You will eat differently on training days and rest days'

Why do I eat this way?

My post-workout carbohydrate-refuel meal structure is very effective for fat loss. Your body stores carbohydrates in the liver and muscles as glycogen and, after a workout, these are depleted, so you need to 'refuel' and top up those stores after training. When you consume carbohydrates, they are broken down into sugars and this increases your blood sugar levels, causing the pancreas to release insulin. Remember, this is a good thing post-workout as insulin shuttles the nutrients from your meal into your muscles quickly, so they can get to work repairing and rebuilding.

Whenever you're not working intensively, your body uses mainly fats for fuel. This is why you will reduce your carbohydrates on rest days and increase your fat intake. At first you might struggle to make this change. Psychologically you may feel like you are low on energy, but don't forget you are still providing your body with energy – just from fats instead of carbs. You will soon adjust to it, so persevere. And remember, you are eating to stay lean.

What meals should I choose?

The training plan is flexible and all meals are interchangeable. This means you could have protein pancakes for breakfast or dinner, depending on when you train. Just remember that you are 'earning' those carbs during your workout, so you must always choose a carbohydrate-refuel meal afterwards, regardless of how late you train.

If there is a recipe you want to try, but you don't like a certain ingredient, such as onions or peppers, simply swap it for something similar that you do enjoy. The same goes with the protein – for example, if you don't like beef mince, you can always use turkey mince.

I've included a few treats in the book but these should only be eaten once or twice a week and only after a workout.

Alcohol and fat loss

I'm always very honest and realistic with my clients when it comes to drinking alcohol. I never tell them to cut it out completely, as this is a personal choice for them to make. I just remind them that the less booze they drink, the leaner they will get. Put simply, alcohol puts the brakes on fat loss, as it interferes with the normal metabolic pathways, including fat-burning, in the body.

> 'ALCOHOL PUTS THE BRAKES ON FAT LOSS'

In addition to alcohol preventing you from burning fat, it also contributes a significant amount to your daily intake of calories. It's very easy to drink a lot of calories from alcohol without realizing it, and this can have a big knock-on effect on your training and nutrition the following day. With a hangover, you are not likely to want to train or to eat particularly well – personally, I'll eat everything in sight when hungover, including tubs and tubs of ice cream.

Ultimately you need to find your own balance, but if you really are serious about getting lean and transforming your body, then you will need to sacrifice a few nights out on the booze. Alcohol could well be the one thing holding you back from achieving the body you want.

Hydration

Most people underestimate the importance of hydration for fat loss. Almost two thirds of the human body is made up of water, and it is involved in everything from removing waste and lubricating joints to regulating body temperature. It also aids metabolism, so consumption of water is vital to maximize your body's fat burning ability. As a general rule, I recommend drinking between 2 and 4 litres of water per day. This may seem like a lot, but it really will work wonders for your body inside and out. If you don't enjoy drinking plain water, try adding some fresh mint, lemon or lime for a bit of flavour.

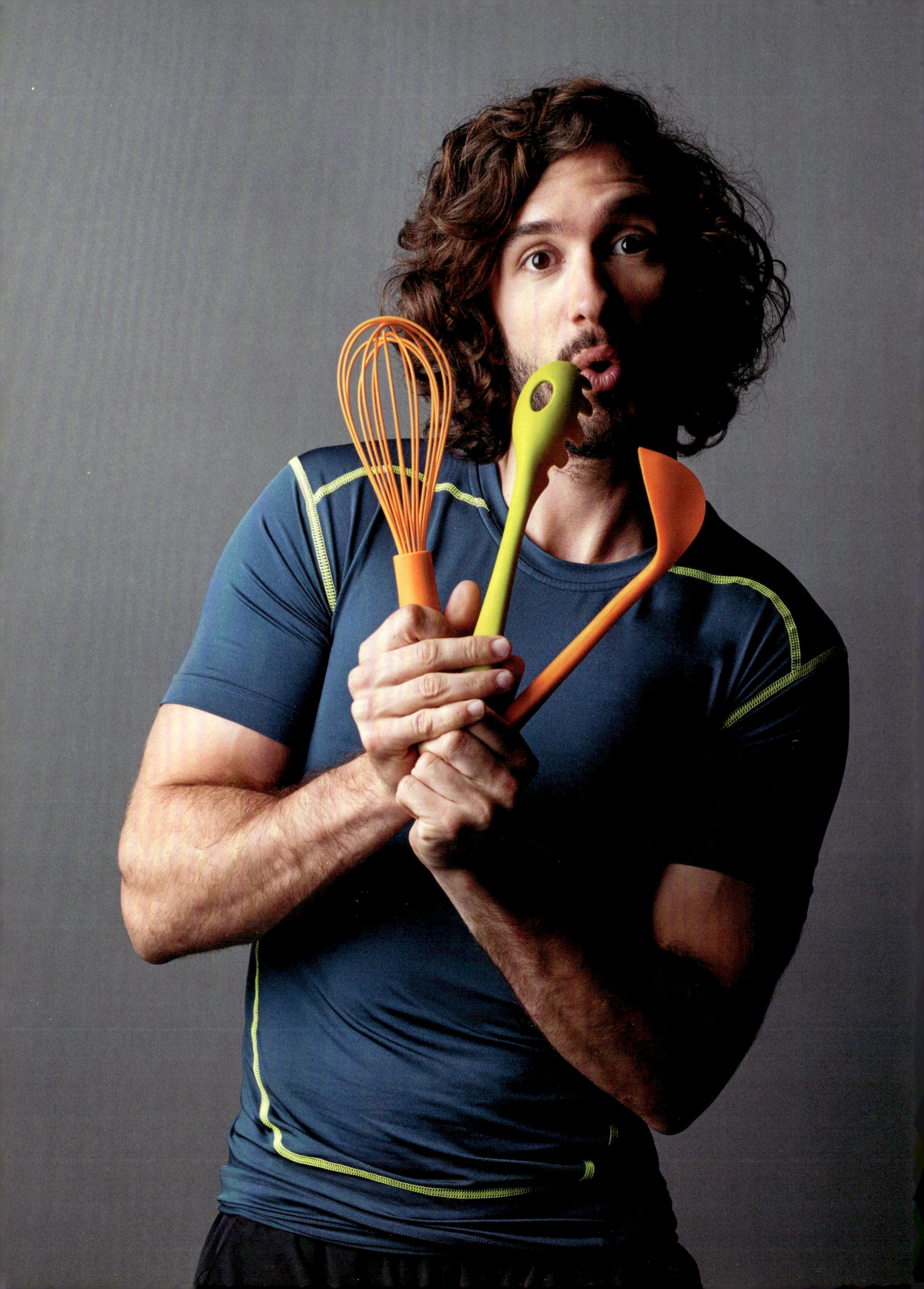

2

GETTING STARTED

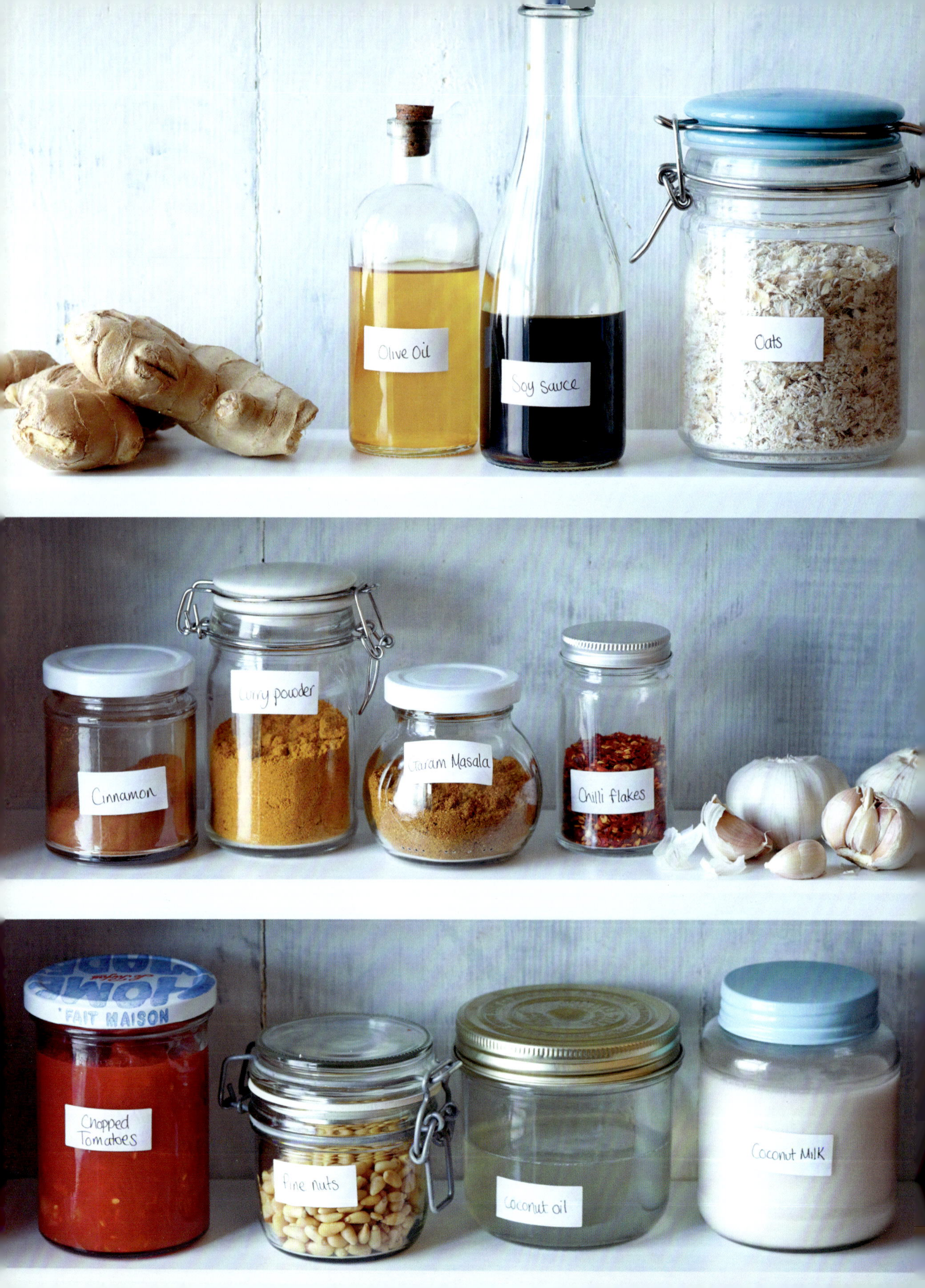
Olive Oil
Soy sauce
Oats
Curry powder
Cinnamon
Garam Masala
Chilli flakes
FAIT MAISON
Chopped Tomatoes
Pine nuts
Coconut oil
Coconut Milk

GETTING STARTED

> No more low calories, zero carbs or low fat for you

Hopefully you now have a better understanding of macronutrients and how you are going to use them to fuel your body to get lean. No more low calories, zero carbs or low fat for you! You are going to eat lots of tasty food, feel full of energy every day, and really give your body a chance to transform.

STEP 1: PLAN LIKE A WINNER

Planning your meals and workouts into the week ahead is the first step for success. You may not be able to follow it 100%, as things will inevitably pop up during the week that are beyond your control. That's life, but it's still important to set yourself daily goals: if you can only manage 3 workouts per week, then that's what you should put in your plan. Keep it realistic and achievable, as small daily wins will increase your motivation to follow your plan.

Start by writing down your workouts and meals into a table like mine on page 214. This will allow you to schedule time for your workouts and also create a shopping list ready for when you prep your meals.

STEP 2:
PREPPING LIKE A BOSS

> I just prep my meals a day or two in advance and keep them in the fridge

Now you have planned like a winner it's time to get your food shopping done and get prepping like a boss. This means spending a couple of hours in the kitchen on a weekend to set yourself up for success. It may seem like a hassle to begin with, but you will get quicker and more organized, and soon it will become an easy habit for you. It's a great feeling to know exactly what you are fuelling your body with, and it means you can avoid buying junk food on the go when you get hungry. You can leave the house with your lunch sorted and your dinner all ready to go, so that after a long day at work or a late session at the gym, you can just stroll in, reheat your meal and refuel your body quickly.

The busier your lifestyle and job is, the further in advance you will need to prep. Some people like to cook and freeze their meals for a week ahead. I personally prefer to eat a bit fresher, so I just prep my meals a day or two in advance and keep them in the fridge. I then either eat them cold or reheat them in the microwave or oven. There is no right or wrong way to do this. Just keep it as stress-free as possible and make it fit your lifestyle – that way you're more likely to stick to it and form good habits.

STEP 3:
GET STOCKED UP!

Now you know how to prep like a boss, you need a few essential tools and ingredients to start putting your plans into action:

1. Food scales – to weigh your ingredients and maintain good portion control
2. Food storage containers – to store and organize all your tasty meals for the week ahead
3. A decent wok and pan – there's nothing worse than a bad wok, so invest in a good one
4. Store cupboard essentials – some core ingredients in the cupboard or fridge, so you don't get caught out

5. A refillable water bottle – to ensure you stay hydrated at all times and can keep track of your water intake each day.

STORE CUPBOARD ESSENTIALS

Garam masala
Curry powder
Fresh root ginger
Ground cinnamon
Garlic
Chilli flakes
Pine nuts
Tinned tomatoes
Oats
Light soy sauce
Olive oil
Coconut oil
Coconut milk

THROW AWAY THE SAD STEP!

I call bathroom scales the sad step because that's exactly what they are: you stand on them every day, and then feel sad when the numbers aren't moving in the right direction. This often results in people losing motivation, bingeing on junk food or quitting a plan altogether. I don't want you to be concerned with the numbers any more.

> **'I don't want you to be concerned with the numbers any more'**

The truth is, when it comes to hitting your health and fitness goals, the sad step is the worst measure of success you can possibly get and it's time you threw it out the window. Because no matter how hard you train, or how well you eat, scales cannot measure some of the most important things when it comes to your body, health and wellbeing.

Things the sad step CANNOT measure:

- Your fitness levels
- Your energy levels
- Your strength
- Changes in your body composition
- Your sense of achievement
- Your confidence
- Your happiness

The best motivational tool for measuring your progress is taking photos of your body. My advice is to take some photos at the end of each month: these will show your true progress and keep you motivated to carry on, even when the mirror starts playing tricks on you and you convince yourself you haven't changed.

> 'Fat loss is a journey not a race'

GO GET LEAN

Once you've got your meals and workouts planned, you can start your journey to a fitter, stronger and leaner version of yourself. Remember, fat loss is a journey not a race, so be patient and be consistent.

LET'S GET SOCIAL

If you want to see more recipes or share your meals and progress with me, post and tag your pics with the hashtag #Leanin15 on Twitter, Instagram and Facebook @thebodycoach.

For more HIIT workouts, check out my YouTube channel TheBodyCoachTV.

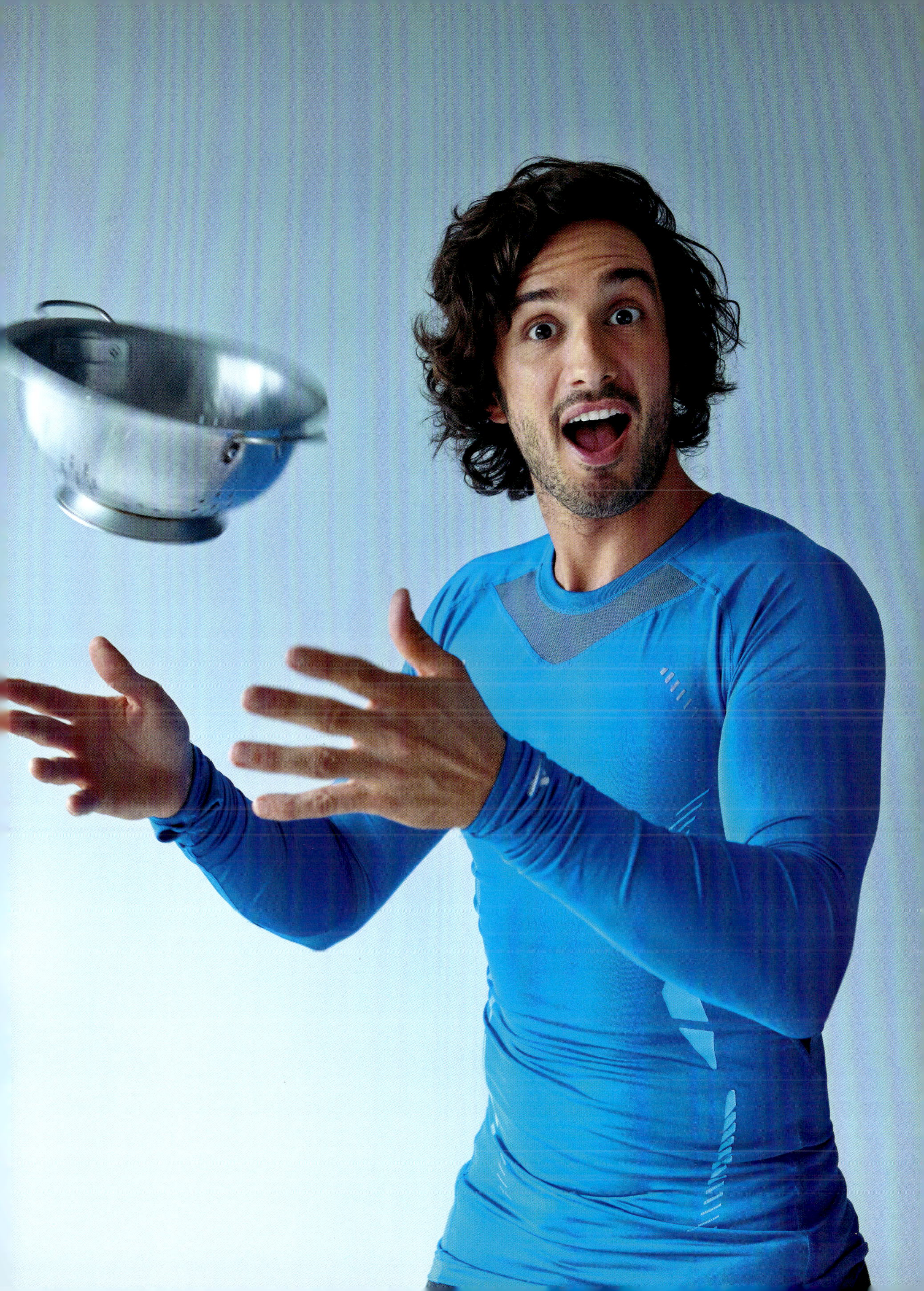

3

REDUCED-CARBOHYDRATE RECIPES

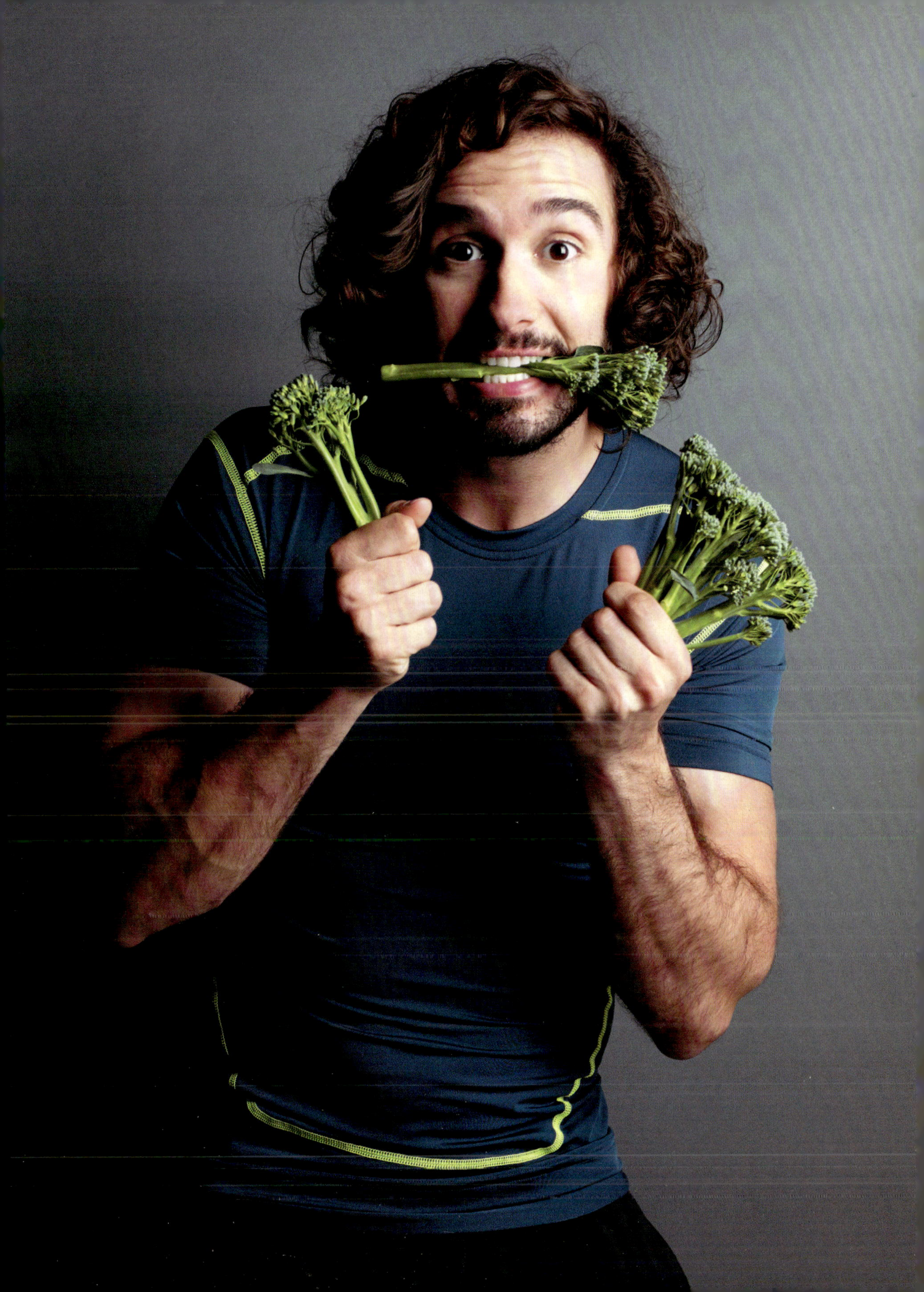

NUT AND MANGO SMOOTHIE

SERVES 1

This fruity smoothie is ideal for a last-minute breakfast on the go. With healthy fats and a scoop of protein powder, this is way better for you than any bowl of boxed cereal. Try not to get into the habit of having smoothies every day, though. As I always say, real food wins over dust every time.

INGREDIENTS

- 125g sliced mango
- 2 tbsp almond or cashew butter
- handful of ice cubes
- handful of raspberries
- 2 tbsp full-fat Greek yoghurt
- 1 scoop (30g) vanilla or strawberry protein powder
- 100ml almond milk

METHOD

Place all the ingredients in a blender and blend until smooth.

★ TOP TIP

Warning! Don't go nuts with your nuts. While they are a great source of protein, fibre and essential fats, nuts also contain lots of calories. It's very easy to crack open a 200g bag and finish the lot without feeling full. But remember every gram of fat contains 9 kcal, so overeating nuts will not help with your fat loss. I recommend a snack portion of 25–30g. Also, try to get a variety of different nuts as they contain different vitamins. Almonds, walnuts and cashews are my personal favourites.

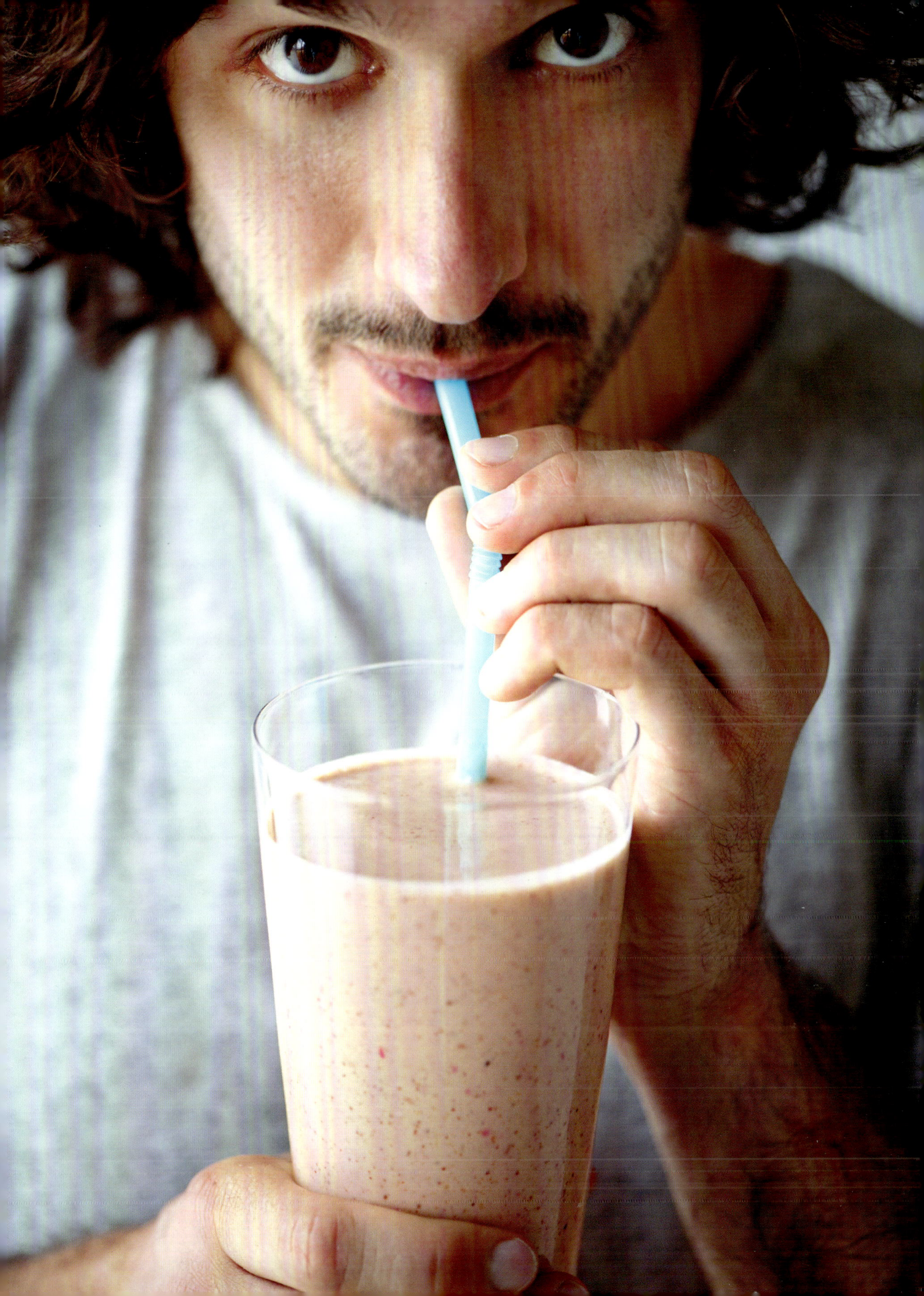

FATS-ME-UP SMOOTHIE

SERVES 1

Here's another tasty low-carb smoothie you can drink on the go. The almond milk and avocado provide you with some healthy fats for fuel, but feel free to add a scoop of your favourite protein too for an extra boost. Make sure you use a soft, ripe avocado for this.

INGREDIENTS

juice of 2 limes
200ml almond milk
handful of blackberries
handful of blueberries
½ avocado, roughly chopped
3 tbsp full-fat Greek yoghurt
1 tbsp honey

METHOD

Throw everything into a blender and blitz until smooth.

★ TOP TIP

The avocado is a nutritional hero in my eyes, with a long list of health benefits. It's a great source of monounsaturated oleic acid, which research has shown reduces levels of bad LDL cholesterol at the same time as increasing levels of the more beneficial HDL cholesterol. That means this little rascal is actually good for your heart.

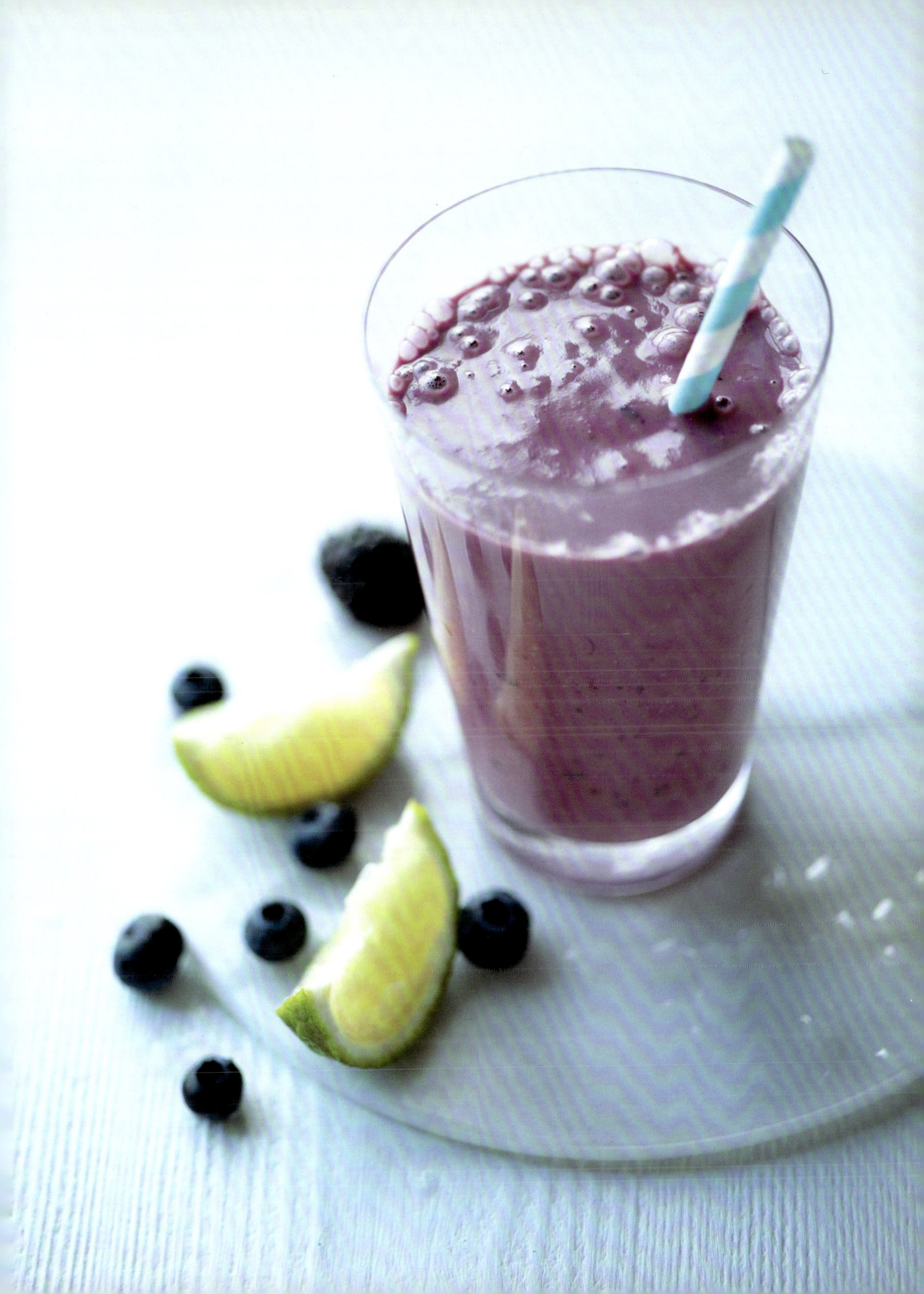

SERVES 1

CINNAMON REDUCED-CARB OATMEAL

INGREDIENTS

- 22g chia seeds
- 22g golden flaxseed meal
- 40g finely shredded unsweetened coconut
- 30g oats – rolled or steel-cut, not instant
- ¾ tsp ground cinnamon
- 300ml almond milk, plus a little extra if needed
- 3 tbsp full-fat Greek yoghurt

I always like to encourage people to think outside the cereal box at breakfast but there's nothing wrong with a good bowl of oats. The added chia and flaxseeds in this meal provide a dose of those all-important and essential omega-3 fatty acids. This one will leave you feeling full and energized until lunch.

METHOD

Place all the ingredients except the yoghurt in a small saucepan and cook gently over low heat for 5–6 minutes until you're happy with the consistency – add a little more almond milk if the oatmeal gets too thick.

Transfer to a bowl, dollop the yoghurt on top and serve.

★ **TOP TIP**

Flaxseeds (also called linseeds) are a rich source of micronutrients, dietary fibre, vitamin B1 and an omega-3 fatty acid called alpha-linoleic acid (ALA). So if you don't enjoy eating oily fish, try to get flaxseeds into your diet more often.

SERVES 1

GO-GO-GREEN SMOOTHIE

INGREDIENTS

- 175ml coconut water
- 2 tbsp almond butter
- 25g fresh wheatgrass (or 5g powdered)
- 1 scoop (30g) vanilla protein powder
- 1 apple, cored and roughly chopped
- 20g flaxseeds
- handful of baby spinach leaves
- handful of ice cubes

Mums always tell us to eat our greens, so here you go. If you're not a big fan of leafy green veg, then this is the perfect opportunity for you to smash them in. Wheatgrass is very good for you – but, just like Marmite, it's a love or hate kind of thing. If you don't enjoy it, just leave it out and add more spinach or some kale instead.

METHOD

Put all the ingredients in a blender and blend on high for 1 minute or until the smoothie has reached your desired texture.

CAULIFLOWER COUSCOUS CHICKEN SALAD

SERVES 2

In my opinion, cauliflower is underrated and underused. It's extremely nutritious and full of goodness. Use this recipe as a basis to experiment with other flavour combinations – try it with smoked mackerel instead of chicken, for example. If you want a warm dish, just microwave the cauliflower on its own and then add the other ingredients.

MAKE AHEAD

INGREDIENTS

- 1 cauliflower, broken into florets
- 4 tbsp pomegranate seeds
- 5 sundried tomatoes, roughly chopped
- 2 jarred red peppers, roughly chopped
- 2 tbsp walnut oil or olive oil
- 4 tbsp walnuts, roughly chopped
- ½ bunch of chives, finely sliced
- ½ bunch of parsley, leaves only, roughly chopped
- large handful of baby spinach leaves
- 400g cooked skinless chicken breast (deli chicken is perfect)
- juice of 1 lemon

METHOD

Place the cauliflower florets in a food processor and pulse until they have a couscous-like texture.

Tip your cauliflower couscous into a large bowl and add all the other ingredients except the chicken and lemon juice. Mix the whole lot thoroughly.

Pile up your couscous on plates, then top with the cooked chicken and a good squeeze of lemon juice.

CHEESY CHORIZO CHICKEN AND SPINACH

SERVES 1

This is pretty much the simplest dish you can imagine. And melted cheese is sooooo satisfying! You can also try this with prawns or turkey mince for a change, if you like.

INGREDIENTS

½ tbsp coconut oil
75g chorizo, finely diced
½ red onion, diced
1 x 240g skinless chicken breast fillet, cut into 1cm slices
salt and pepper
4 cherry tomatoes, sliced in half
3 big fistfuls of baby spinach leaves
1 ball of mozzarella, torn into chunks
20g pine nuts

METHOD

Heat the coconut oil in a large frying pan over a medium to high heat. Add the chorizo and fry for a minute. Add the onion and fry for another minute.

Increase the heat to maximum and add the chicken, along with a generous pinch of both salt and pepper. Stir-fry for about 3 minutes, by which time the chicken should be almost completely cooked through.

Throw in the cherry tomatoes and cook for a minute or until they just begin to collapse. Toss in the spinach and stir through until fully wilted.

Use a wooden spoon to make little pockets in the chicken and vegetable mixture, then drop in small chunks of the mozzarella. Turn off the heat and let the mozzarella melt before spooning the whole delicious lot onto a plate and scattering over the pine nuts.

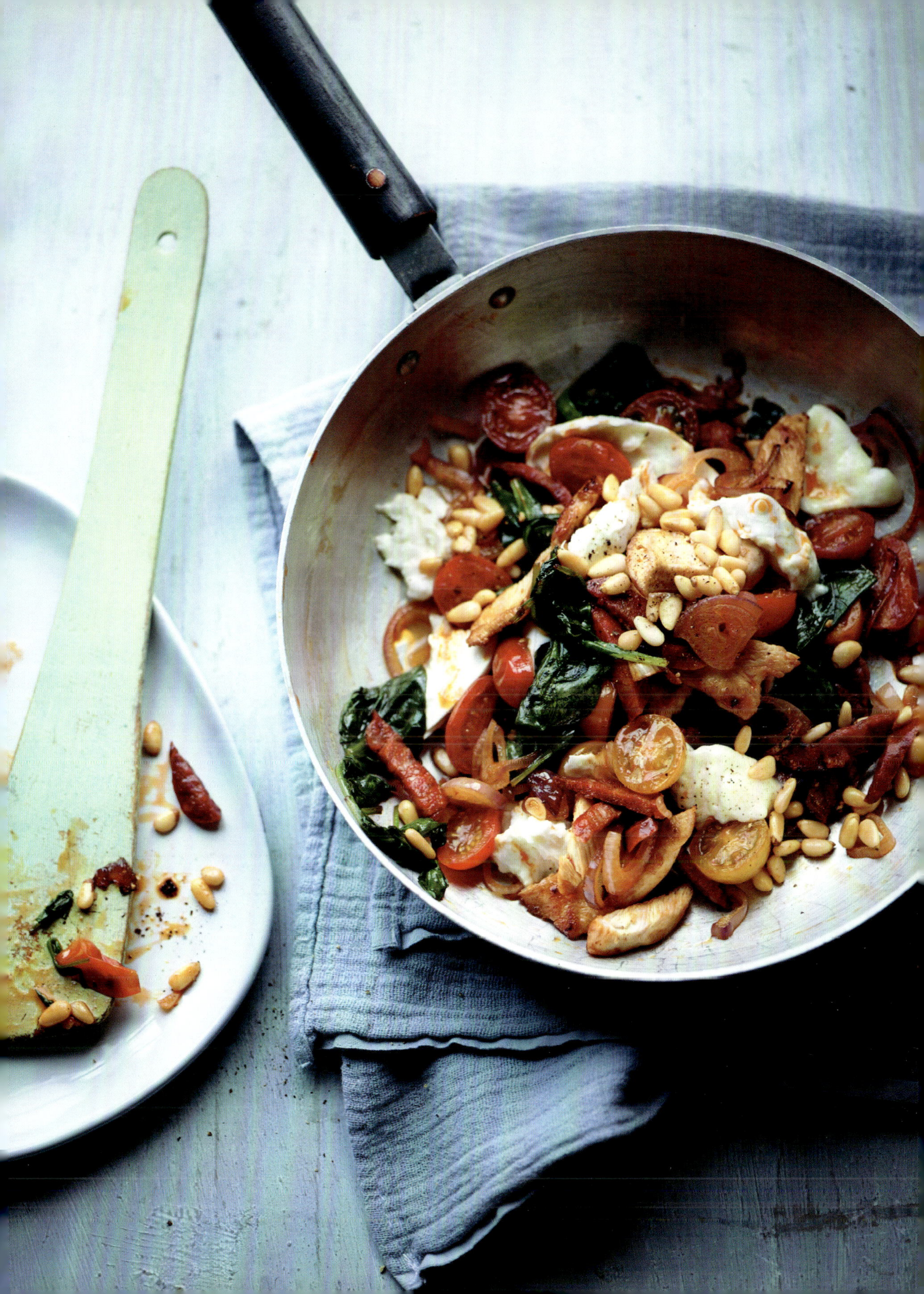

CHICKEN WITH CREAMY WILD MUSHROOM AND TARRAGON SAUCE

SERVES 2

GOOD TO FREEZE

INGREDIENTS

2 x 225g skinless chicken breast fillets
1 tbsp olive oil
1 clove garlic, finely chopped
300g mixed mushrooms – I like chestnut and oyster
splash of white wine
2 large handfuls of baby spinach leaves
150ml double cream
½ bunch of tarragon, leaves only, roughly chopped
salt and pepper

This old-school classic really hits the spot: it's so full of flavour, and poaching the chicken keeps it nice and moist. Most supermarkets now stock some great wild mushrooms, so be adventurous and get some exotic-looking ones.

METHOD

Bring a large saucepan of water to the boil, then slide in the chicken. Lower the heat until the water is just 'burping' and not vigorously boiling. Let the chicken cook for 12 minutes, by which time it should be fully cooked through.

Meanwhile, heat the oil in a large frying pan over a medium to high heat. Add the garlic and cook for about 30 seconds. Roughly chop any larger mushrooms and throw them into the pan, to give them a head start for a minute or two before adding the rest of the mushrooms and cooking for another minute.

Increase the heat to maximum, then pour in the white wine and let it bubble away to almost nothing. Drop in the spinach and stir until wilted. Pour in the double cream, then bring to the boil and simmer for 1 minute. Add the chopped tarragon and remove the pan from the heat.

Check that the chicken is cooked by slicing into the thickest part of the breast: the meat should be white all the way through and the juices should run clear, not pink. Remove to a plate, draining off as much liquid as possible. Season with salt and pepper, then place on two plates and pour over the delicious creamy sauce.

★ Serve with a big portion of your favourite greens such as spinach, kale, broccoli, mange tout or green beans.

SERVES 1

MAKE AHEAD

GOOD TO FREEZE

(if freezing, increase the amount of stock to 150ml)

SUPER-SPEEDY BEEF STROGANOFF

Fillet steak is the best cut for this dish, but it is expensive, so if you're on a budget opt for sirloin or rump. If you love steak then this one is a real winner.

INGREDIENTS

- 2 tsp coconut oil
- 2 shallots, finely sliced
- 5 chestnut mushrooms, roughly chopped
- 300g fillet steak, cut into 1cm thick strips
- salt and pepper
- 2 tsp smoked paprika
- 75ml beef stock
- 125ml soured cream
- ½ bunch of parsley, leaves only, roughly chopped – optional
- juice of 1 lemon

METHOD

Melt the coconut oil in a frying pan over a high heat. Add the shallots and mushrooms and fry, stirring regularly, for 2–3 minutes or until the shallots have softened and the mushrooms have taken on a little colour.

Add the beef, along with a generous pinch of both salt and pepper, and stir-fry for 1–2 minutes. Sprinkle in the smoked paprika and toss to lightly coat everything with the spice.

Pour in the beef stock – it will bubble up quickly – then turn the heat right down and stir in the soured cream. Take the pan off the heat, then add the parsley, if using, and a generous squeeze of lemon juice. Serve and enjoy.

★ Serve with a big portion of your favourite greens such as spinach, kale, broccoli, mange tout or green beans.

SERVES 1

FRESH TUNA NIÇOISE

I love using fresh tuna for this salad, as it tastes amazing, but if you'd rather use tinned tuna, that's fine too. This makes a great packed lunch to carry to work.

MAKE AHEAD

INGREDIENTS

- 1 egg
- 75g green beans, trimmed
- ½ tbsp coconut oil
- 1 x 300g tuna fillet
- salt and pepper
- 2 tbsp pre-cooked puy lentils
- large handful of baby spinach leaves
- 1 tbsp sundried tomatoes (about 6)
- 20g walnuts, roughly chopped
- 1 tbsp olive oil
- 2 tsp balsamic or sherry vinegar

METHOD

Bring a medium-sized saucepan of water to the boil before carefully lowering in the egg. Boil for 8 minutes, then drop in the green beans and simmer for a further minute.

Meanwhile, heat the coconut oil in a frying pan over a medium to high heat. Carefully lay in the tuna and fry for 1 minute on each side. This will give you rare tuna – if you like it more cooked, fry it for a further minute on each side. Remove the tuna from the pan, season and leave to rest while you put the rest of the salad together.

Drain the egg and beans in a sieve or colander, then run under cold water until cool enough to handle. Peel the egg and slice in half. Put the beans, lentils, spinach, sundried tomatoes, walnuts, olive oil and vinegar into a bowl, along with a generous pinch of salt and pepper. Gently toss all the ingredients together, then transfer to a plate.

Top the salad with the tuna, sliced if you like, and the egg.

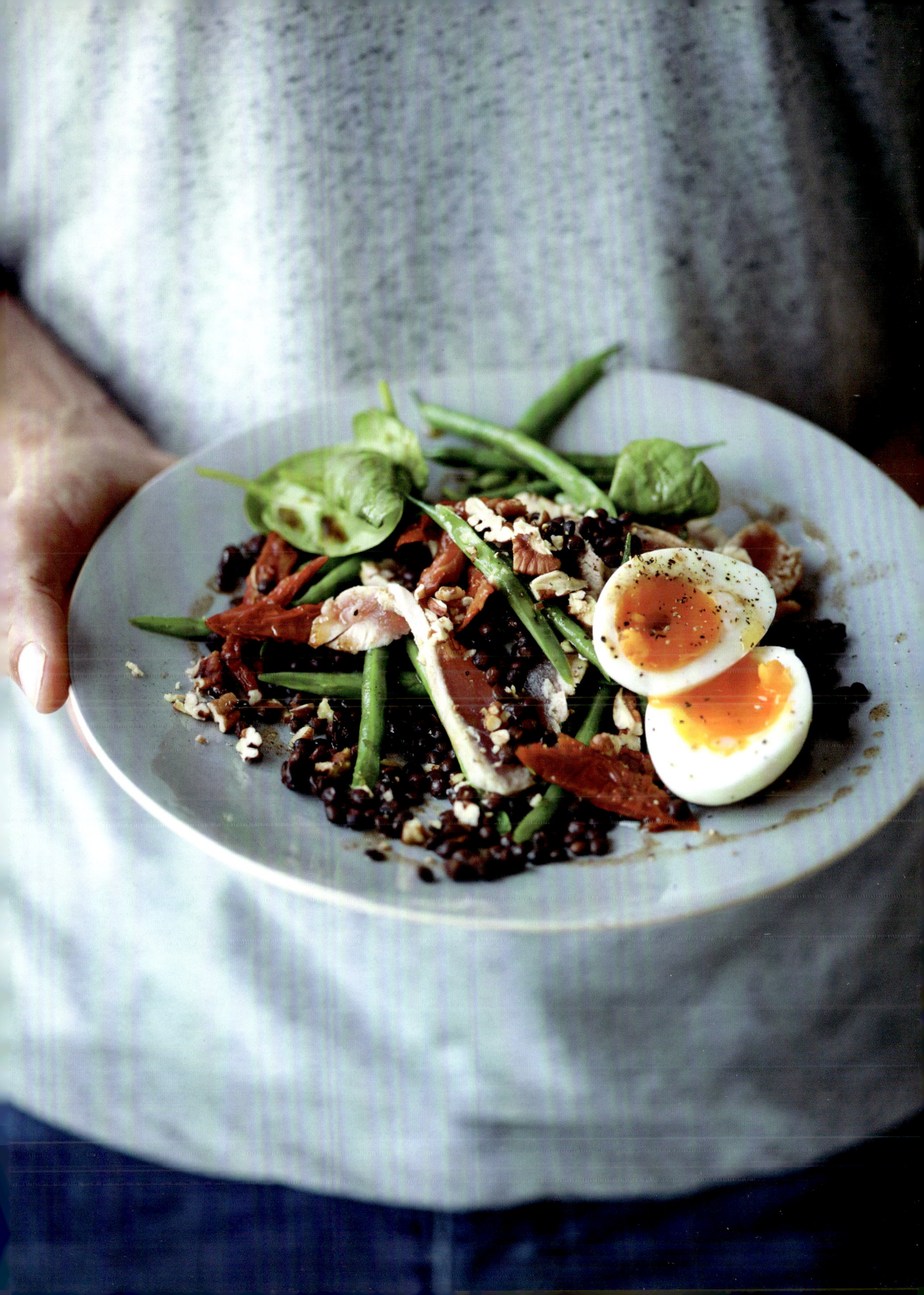

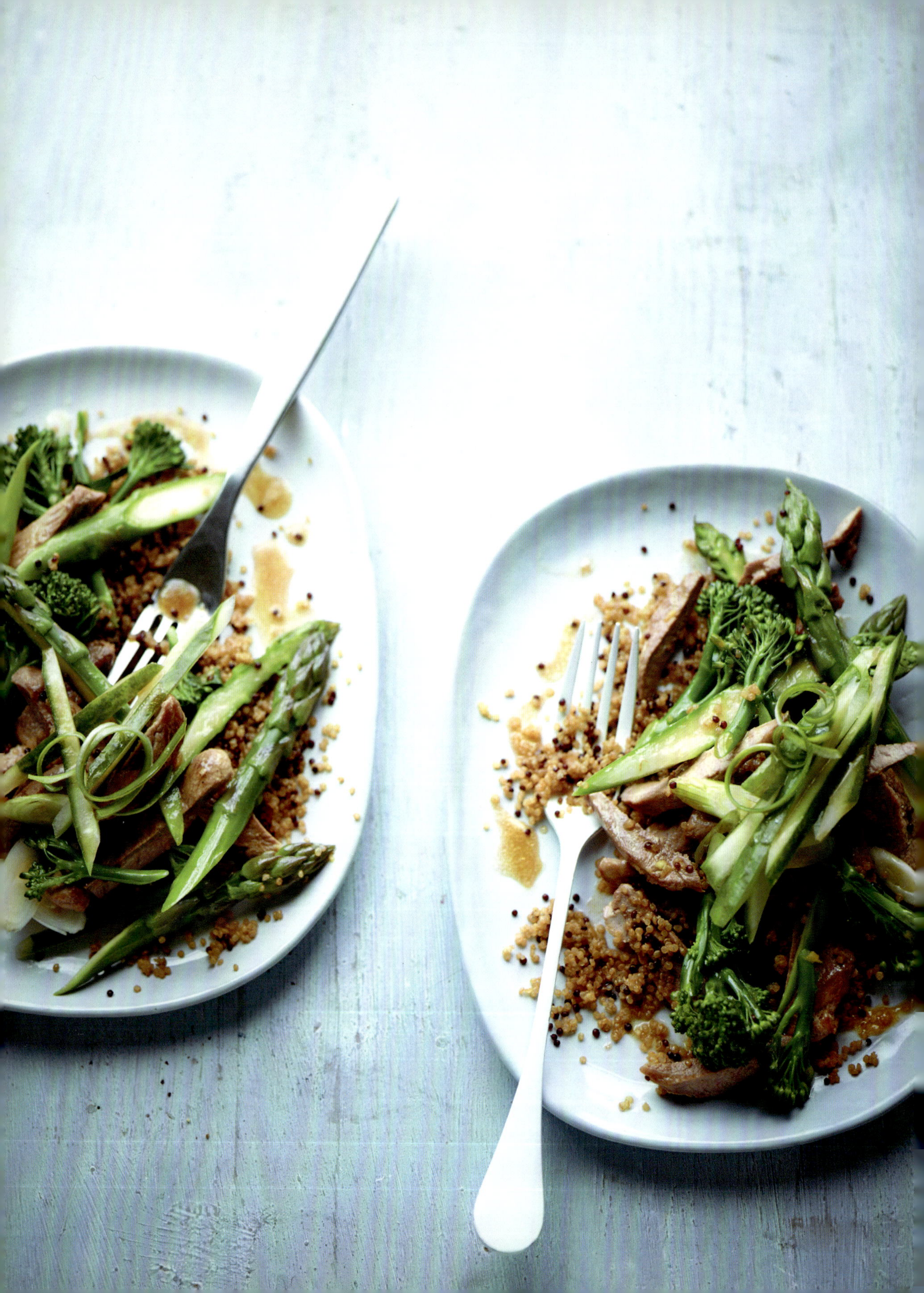

ASIAN DUCK SALAD

SERVES 1

MAKE AHEAD

INGREDIENTS

5 spears of asparagus
4 midget trees (tender-stem broccoli), any bigger stalks sliced in half lengthways
½ tbsp coconut oil
1 x 250g duck breast fillet, sliced into 1cm thick strips
2cm ginger, finely chopped
1 tbsp light soy sauce
2 tsp sesame oil
2 tbsp ready-cooked quinoa
1 spring onion, finely sliced
¼ cucumber, sliced into thin batons

Duck is a rich and delicious meat that's packed with protein. For the veg, I've gone with asparagus and midget trees (my name for broccoli!), but feel free to improvise. Having fun in the kitchen and mixing it up will help to keep things tasty and vary your nutrients. As you can see, I've doubled the recipe in the picture.

METHOD

Take each asparagus spear in turn and bend it gently until it snaps – it will naturally snap at the point where it becomes tender. Discard the bottom of the spear.

Bring a large saucepan of water to the boil, then drop in the asparagus and the midget trees and simmer for 1½ minutes. Drain in a sieve or colander, then rinse under cold running water.

Melt the coconut oil in a frying pan over a high heat. Add the duck and stir-fry for 30 seconds, then add the ginger and stir-fry for a further minute, by which time the duck should be cooked through. Remove the pan from the heat and stir through the soy sauce and sesame oil.

Place the cooked vegetables in a bowl, then add the quinoa and the duck, along with all its juices. Mix the whole lot together before transferring to a plate and topping with the spring onion and cucumber.

THAI GREEN CURRY

SERVES 4

MAKE AHEAD
GOOD TO FREEZE

INGREDIENTS

- 2 tbsp coconut oil
- 2 star anise
- 1 small aubergine, chopped into small pieces
- 2 tbsp Thai green curry paste
- 1 x 400ml tin of full-fat coconut milk
- handful of baby sweetcorn
- 450g raw king prawns, peeled
- 1–2 tbsp fish sauce
- 3 limes
- ½ bunch of basil, leaves only, roughly chopped
- ½ bunch of coriander, leaves only, roughly chopped
- 1 red chilli, roughly chopped – remove the seeds if you don't like it hot

This tasty classic is my all-time favourite meal. In this version I've suggested prawns, but chicken and pork would work just as well. Bump up the flavour by using full-fat coconut milk, which is packed with good fat. Fish sauce is great to have in the cupboard: it keeps for ages, and even though it smells terrible, it tastes amazing.

METHOD

Melt the coconut oil in a large saucepan over a medium to high heat. Add the star anise and aubergine and fry for 1 minute, then add in the curry paste (store-bought is fine) and half the coconut milk. Stir the paste into the milk, then increase the heat to maximum.

Pour in the rest of the coconut milk, then half-fill the tin with water, slosh it around and pour this into the pan as well. Toss in the sweetcorn, then bring to the boil and simmer for 3 minutes. Drop in the prawns and simmer for a further 2 minutes until they turn pink and are fully cooked.

Take the pan off the heat and chuck in the fish sauce to taste, the juice of 2 of the limes, the herbs and the chilli.

Serve up the curry in bowls, with the last lime cut into quarters for squeezing.

★ TOP TIP

Here's my recipe to make your own Thai green curry paste:

- 4 banana shallots, peeled and chopped
- 4cm galangal, peeled and chopped
- 4 cloves garlic, peeled and chopped
- 2 stalks lemongrass, trimmed and chopped
- 1 tsp cumin seeds
- ½ tsp coriander seeds
- 1 bunch of basil
- 2 bunches of coriander
- 1 tbsp fish sauce
- pinch of grated star anise

Blend the whole lot together using either a little warm water or coconut milk to loosen. You can keep this in an airtight container in the fridge for up to 5 days.

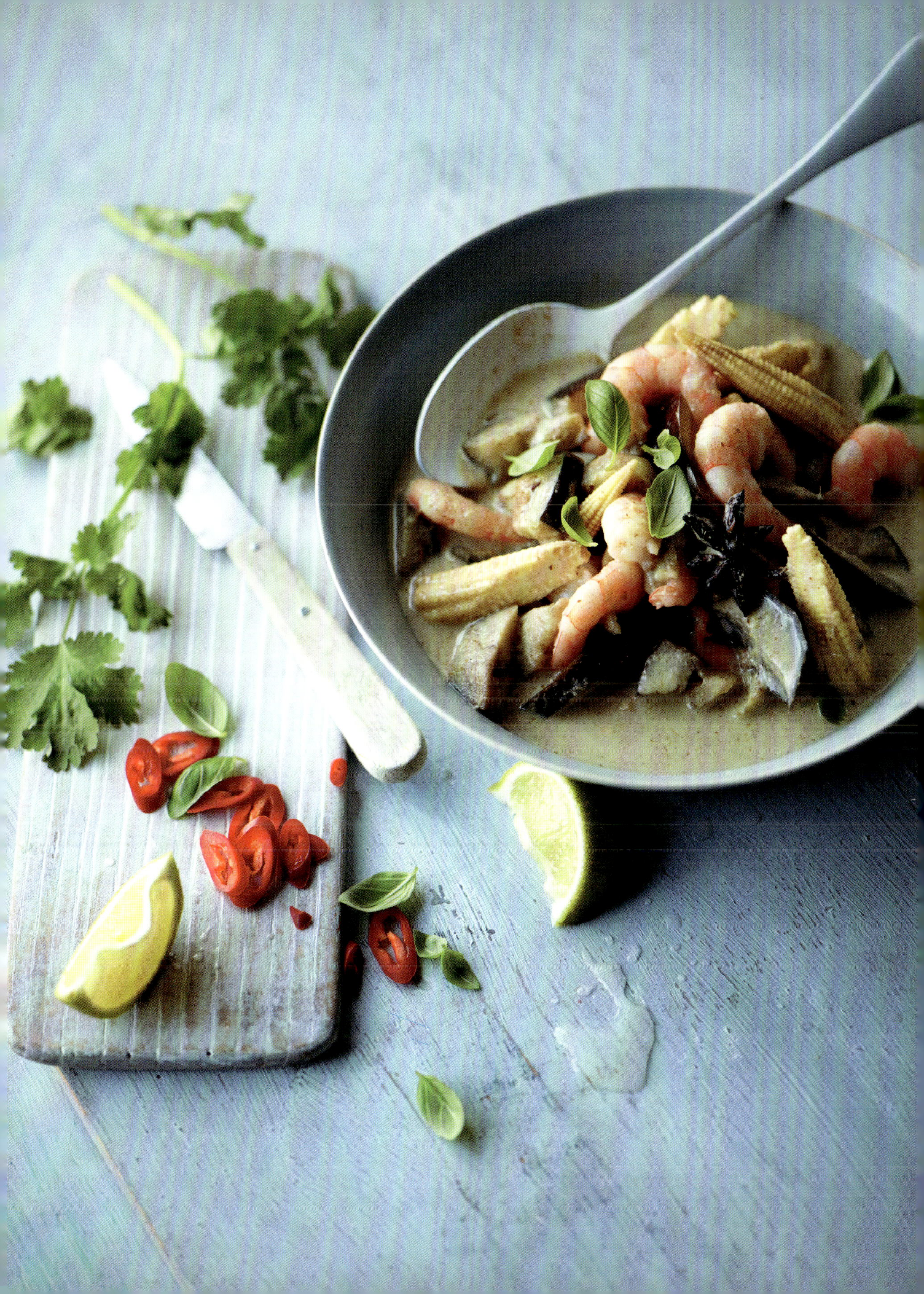

SERVES 1

FRENCH STYLE COD WITH BLACK OLIVES

This is a simple and delicious dish based on a classic French combo. If you're not a fan of cod, you could use any other white fish of your choice.

MAKE AHEAD
GOOD TO FREEZE

INGREDIENTS

- 20g butter
- 2 rashers of smoked streaky bacon, cut into 1cm strips
- ½ red onion, diced
- 1 clove garlic, finely chopped
- 250g cod fillet, skinned and cut into 2cm chunks
- 1 x 400g tin chopped tomatoes
- 8 pitted black olives
- 1 ball of mozzarella, torn into chunks
- 20g pine nuts
- basil leaves, to serve – optional

METHOD

Melt the butter in a large frying pan over a medium to high heat. Add the bacon and onion and fry for 2 minutes or until the onion is starting to soften and the bacon is cooked. Add the garlic and cook for a further 30 seconds.

Drop in the chunks of cod and fry, turning the chunks every now and then, for 2 minutes. Add the tomatoes and bring to the boil. Reduce the heat to a simmer and cook for 2–3 minutes.

Add the olives and mozzarella, then take the pan off the heat and let the mozzarella melt in the residual heat.

Serve the cod topped with the pine nuts – and the basil leaves, if using.

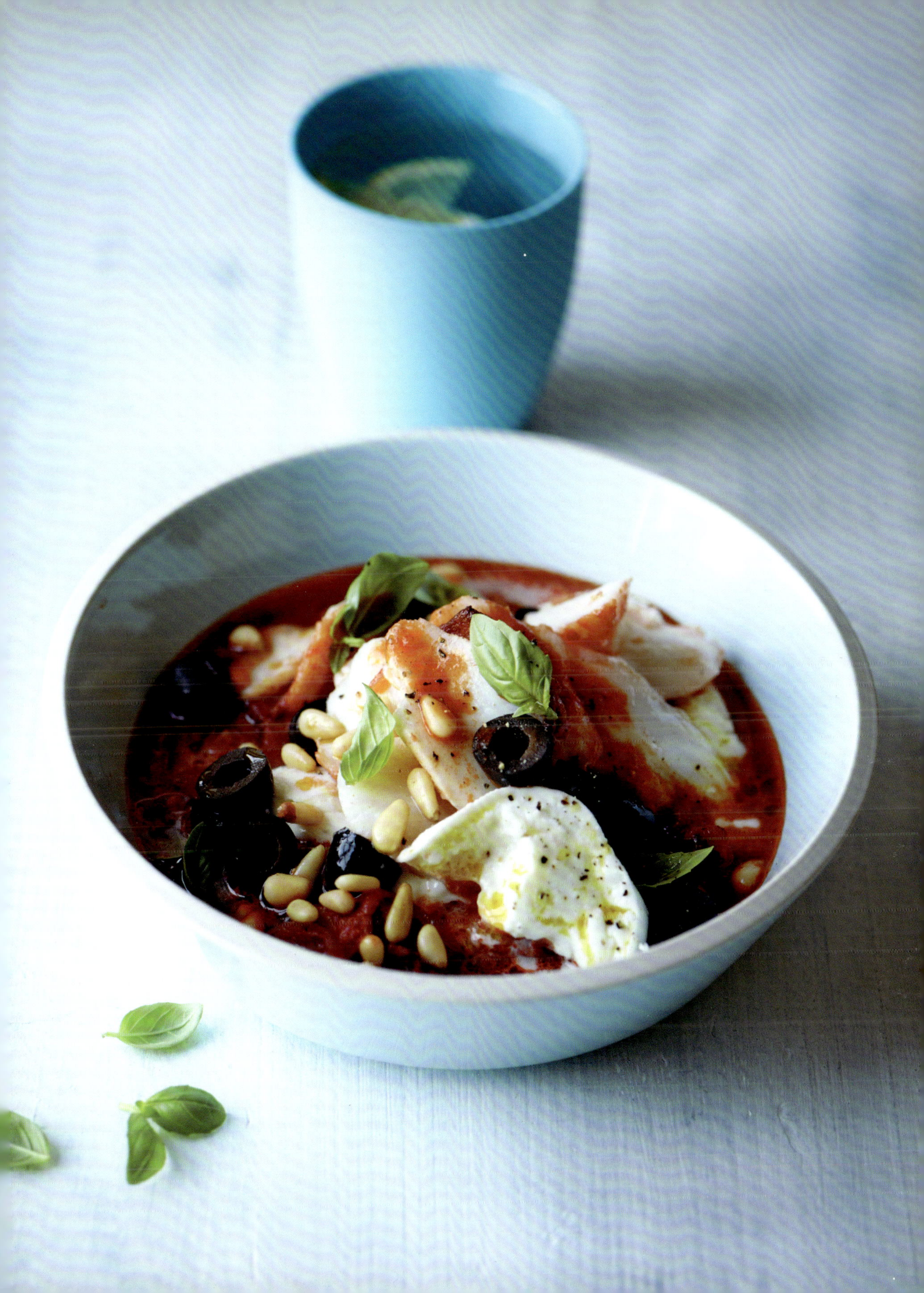

EGGS BAKED IN AVOCADO

SERVES 1

This is becoming a bit of a signature dish for me. I've posted it a few times, and I love seeing people make it at home and share it on Instagram. It contains more healthy fats than you can shake a stick at . . . oh, and it's got bacon too, so you know it's going to taste as good as it looks.

INGREDIENTS

- 4 rashers of smoked back bacon
- 1 ripe avocado
- 2 eggs
- salt and pepper
- 1 red chilli, finely sliced – remove the seeds if you don't like it hot

METHOD

Preheat your grill to maximum, then lay the bacon on the grill pan or a baking tray and slide underneath. Grill for 3 minutes on each side for crispy bacon.

Meanwhile, cut your avocado in half, remove the stone and scoop out a generous tablespoon of flesh from each half to create a hole big enough for the egg. No need to waste the leftover avocado – you can save it to make some guacamole or just eat it on the spot!

Crack an egg into each avocado half, pierce each egg white in a couple of places, season with a little salt and pepper and place on a microwaveable plate. Cook the eggs in 30-second bursts for 2 minutes – this should ensure firm whites, but runny yolks. Leave to stand for 1 minute.

Serve up the baked eggs and avocado with the bacon and a scattering of chilli.

⋆ TOP TIP

To stop the avocados rocking on the plate, slice off a little bit underneath to make a flat base.

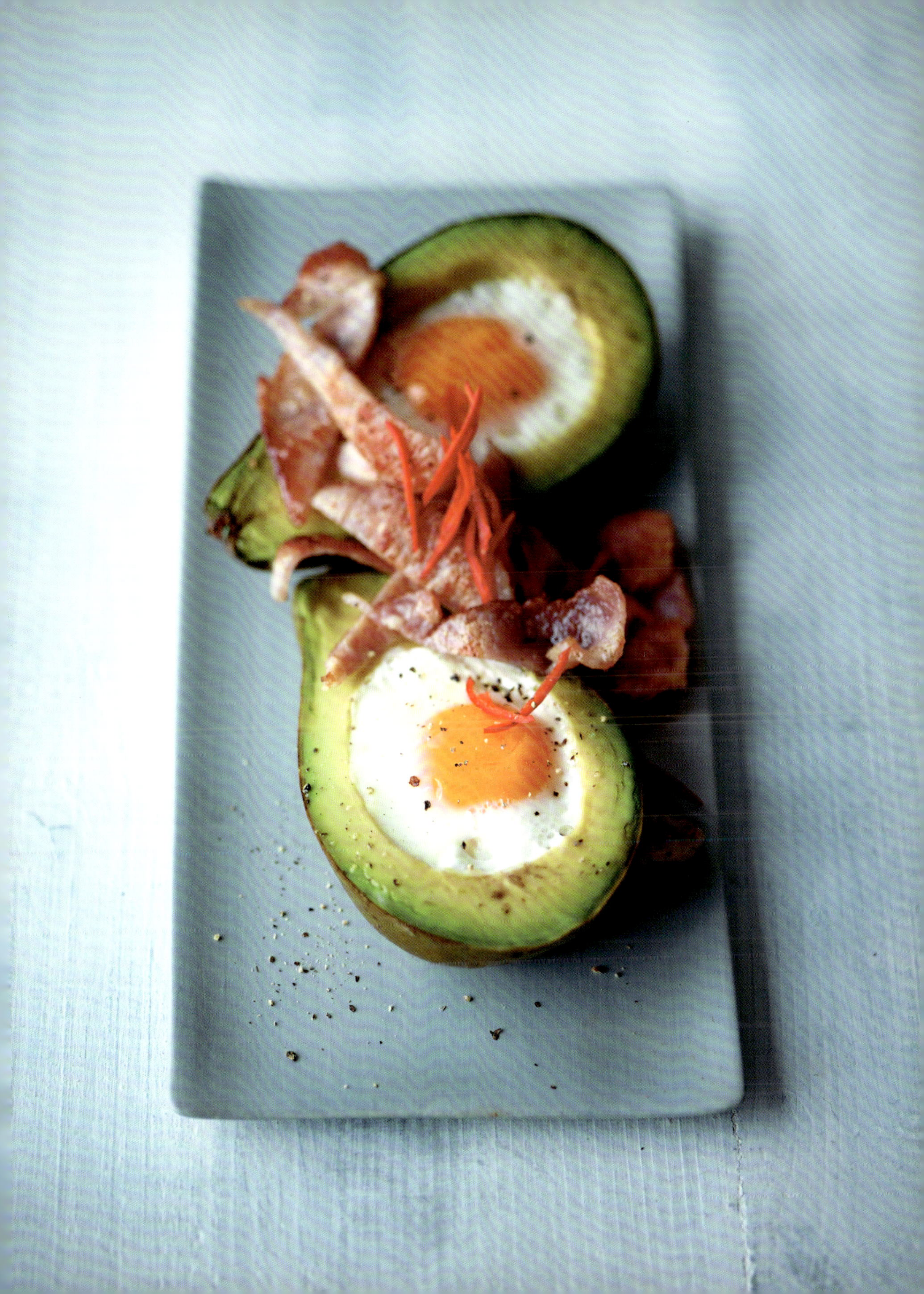

INDIAN SPICED LAMB

SERVES 1

MAKE AHEAD

INGREDIENTS

150g natural yoghurt
2 tbsp ground almonds
2 tsp garam masala
1 tsp smoked paprika
salt and pepper
4 lamb cutlets, about 200g each
large handful of baby spinach leaves
4 cherry tomatoes, halved
¼ cucumber, sliced into batons
½ bunch of coriander, leaves only, roughly chopped
juice of 1 lemon

This is proper dinner-party food! You can see I've doubled the recipe in the picture. Make sure you buy cutlets not chops, because they have a better meat-to-fat ratio. And if you have any leftovers (not likely!), they are delicious the next day, served at room temperature with a big salad.

METHOD

Preheat your grill to maximum and line a baking tray with baking parchment (this is just to make washing up easier).

Place the yoghurt, ground almonds, garam masala and smoked paprika in a bowl, along with a generous amount of salt and pepper. Mix thoroughly.

Smother the lamb cutlets with the spiced yoghurt, then place on the prepared baking tray. Slide the tray under the grill and cook the cutlets for 3–4 minutes on each side, by which time the spiced yoghurt should have browned in a few places.

Meanwhile, make a quick salad by gently tossing the spinach, tomatoes and cucumber together in a bowl. Pile the salad onto a plate.

Remove the lamb cutlets from the grill and leave to rest for 1 or 2 minutes, then sit them on top of the salad. Serve up with a scattering of coriander and a squeeze of lemon juice.

★ Serve with a big portion of your favourite greens such as kale, broccoli, mange tout or green beans.

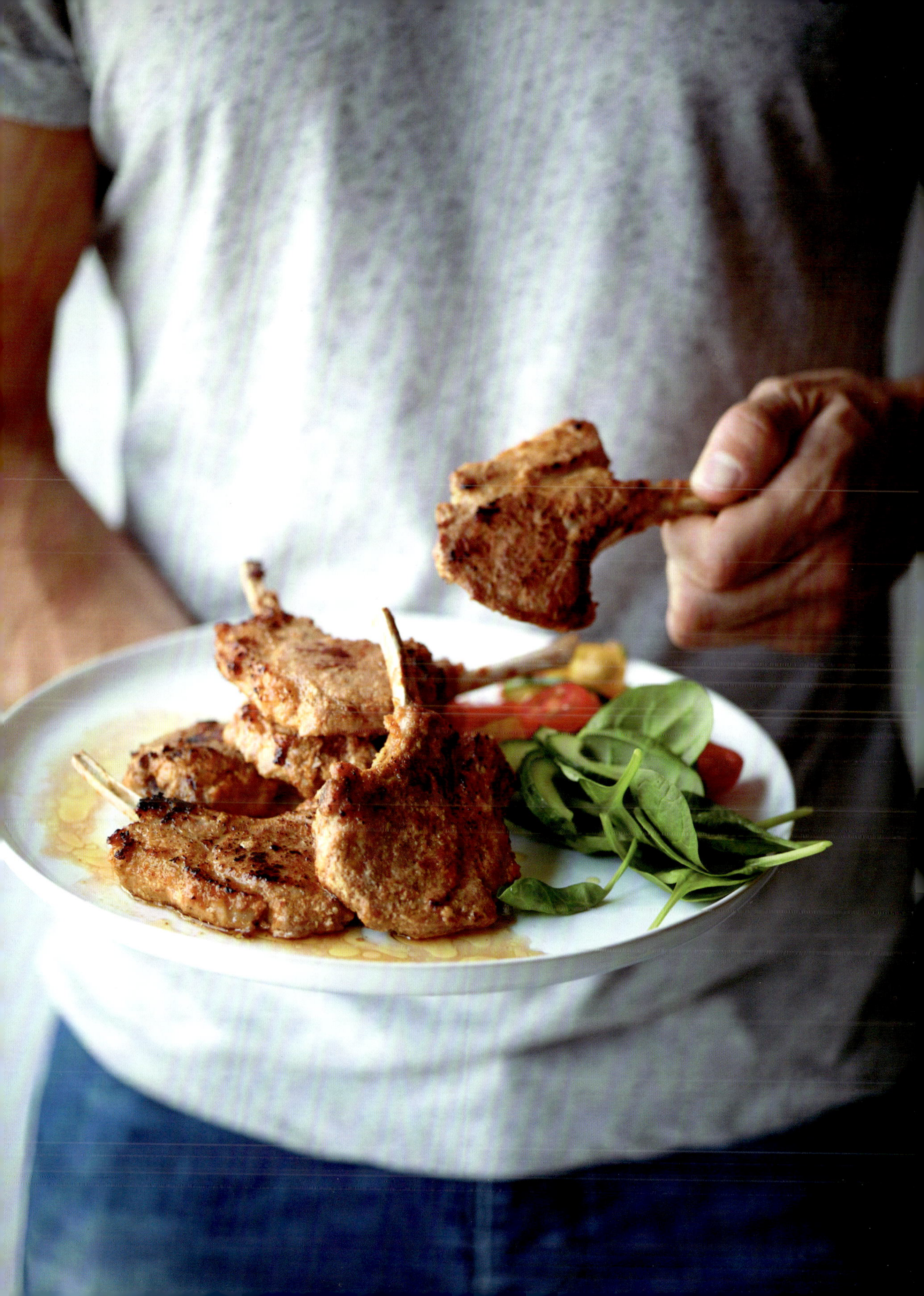

CHICKEN WITH SMOKED PAPRIKA AND ALMONDS

SERVES 1

This is Spanish cooking at its best. I love the combo of almonds and paprika! It's really tasty and so easy to make.

MAKE AHEAD

INGREDIENTS

½ tbsp coconut oil
½ red onion, finely chopped
1 clove garlic, finely chopped
1 red pepper, de-seeded and sliced
2 tsp smoked paprika
1 tsp dried oregano
1 x 240g skinless chicken breast fillet, sliced into 1cm thick strips
5 cherry tomatoes, cut in half
20g blanched almonds
large handful of baby spinach leaves
salt and pepper
juice of 1 lemon

METHOD

Melt the coconut oil in a large frying pan over a medium to high heat. Add the onion, garlic and red pepper and fry, stirring regularly, for 2 minutes or until the vegetables are just starting to soften.

Sprinkle in the smoked paprika and oregano and stir to coat the vegetables, then increase the heat to high. Add the chicken and tomatoes and cook, still stirring regularly, for 3–4 minutes or until the chicken is fully cooked through. Check by slicing into one of the larger pieces to make sure the meat is white all the way through, with no raw pink bits left.

Stir in the almonds and spinach, then cook for a further 2 minutes, or until the spinach has totally wilted.

Plate up your chicken, season generously with salt and pepper, and finish with a squeeze of lemon juice.

★ Serve with a big portion of your favourite greens such as spinach, kale, broccoli, mange tout or green beans.

SALMON WITH CHILLI EDAMAME

SERVES 1

Edamame (soy beans) are now available already podded and frozen, so take advantage of them! This salad is high in omega-3 fatty acids to keep you lean and healthy – and it makes a perfect packed lunch.

MAKE AHEAD

INGREDIENTS

- 1 x 250g salmon fillet, skin on
- 200g frozen edamame (soy beans)
- 1 red chilli, finely diced – remove the seeds if you don't like it hot
- 1 tsp honey
- 2 tsp fish sauce
- 1 tbsp light soy sauce
- 2 tsp sesame oil
- 2 spring onions, finely sliced
- 1 red pepper, de-seeded and sliced
- 25g walnuts
- handful of rocket leaves

METHOD

Bring two saucepans of water to the boil, then slide the salmon fillet into one and drop the edamame into the other. Simmer the edamame for 1½ minutes, then drain in a sieve or colander and rinse under cold running water. Poach the salmon for 12 minutes, or until just cooked through. Using a slotted spoon, carefully lift out the fish and place on a plate. When it is cool enough to handle, peel off the skin.

Meanwhile, mix together the chilli, honey, fish sauce, soy sauce, sesame oil and spring onions to make a dressing.

Tip the edamame into a bowl and add the red pepper, walnuts and rocket. Pour over the dressing and toss the whole lot togethcr.

Place the salad on a plate and serve the salmon on top. This tastes great still warm from the cooking or at room temperature – you decide!

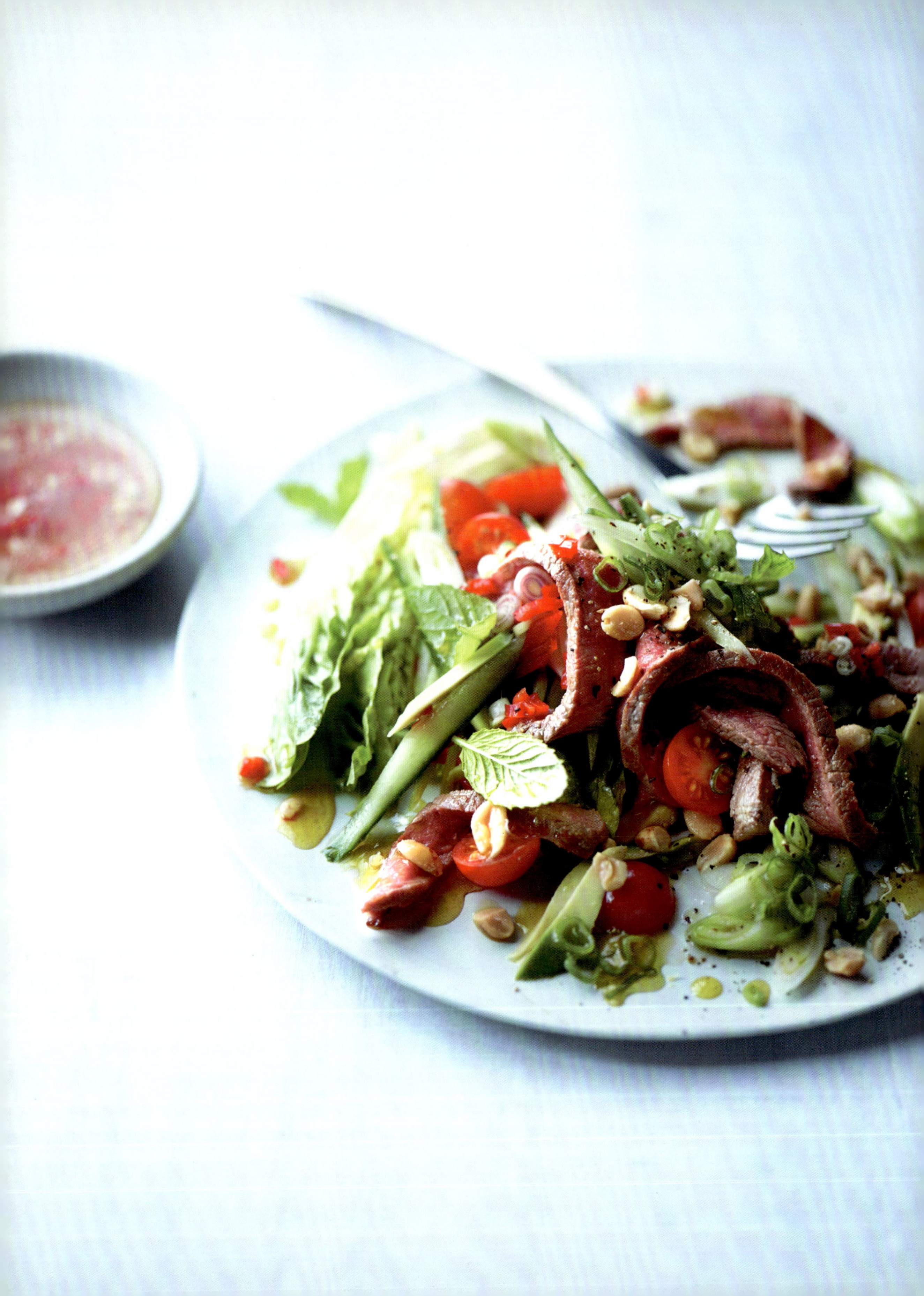

SERVES 1

THAI BEEF SALAD

This is also fantastic with prawns or chicken instead of the beef. You can make up a big batch of the dressing and keep it in the fridge for up to 3 days.

MAKE AHEAD

INGREDIENTS

½ tbsp coconut oil
1 x 250g sirloin steak, trimmed of visible fat
salt and pepper
1 tbsp fish sauce
juice of 2 limes
1 lemongrass stalk, tender white part only, finely sliced
1 red chilli, finely sliced – remove the seeds if you don't like it hot
2 tsp sesame oil
¼ cucumber, sliced into thin batons
2 spring onions, finely sliced
1 avocado, finely sliced
4 cherry tomatoes, cut in half
1 baby gem lettuce, leaves separated
20g peanuts, roughly chopped
mint and coriander leaves, to serve

METHOD

Heat the coconut oil in a frying pan over a high heat. Season the steak all over with salt and pepper. When the oil has melted and is hot, carefully lay the steak in the pan and fry for 2 minutes on each side. When the steak has had its time, transfer it to a plate and leave to rest for 2 minutes.

While the steak is cooking, make a dressing by mixing together the fish sauce, lime juice, lemongrass, chilli and sesame oil in a large bowl. Stir in the cucumber and spring onions, then leave to sit for 2 minutes.

When you are ready to eat, add the avocado, tomatoes and lettuce to the bowl with the dressing, cucumber and spring onions, and gently toss the whole lot together.

Pile up your salad on a plate, slice your steak and place lovingly on the salad, before finishing with the chopped peanuts and roughly torn coriander and mint.

TUNA STEAK WITH SALSA

SERVES 1

If you're not a fan of tinned tuna, then get your hands on a fresh tuna steak. This sort of meal is as good for you as it tastes: the tuna is stacked with protein, and the avocado fuels your body with the healthy fats it needs.

INGREDIENTS

1 x 300g tuna steak
salt and pepper
1 tbsp coconut oil
2 spring onions, finely sliced
2 tbsp tinned black-eyed beans
1 avocado, roughly diced
½ mango (about 100g), roughly diced
1 small tomato, roughly diced
1 tbsp olive oil
juice of 1 lime
¼ bunch of coriander, leaves only, roughly chopped

METHOD

Season the tuna generously with salt and pepper. Melt the oil in a frying pan or griddle pan over a high heat. Gently lay the tuna in the pan and cook for about 2 minutes on each side, or until it's done to your liking. Be careful not to overcook it, as tuna is lean and dries out easily. Transfer the tuna to a plate and leave to rest while you prepare the salsa.

To make the salsa, simply mix together all the remaining ingredients and taste for seasoning.

Spoon the salsa over your perfect tuna steak.

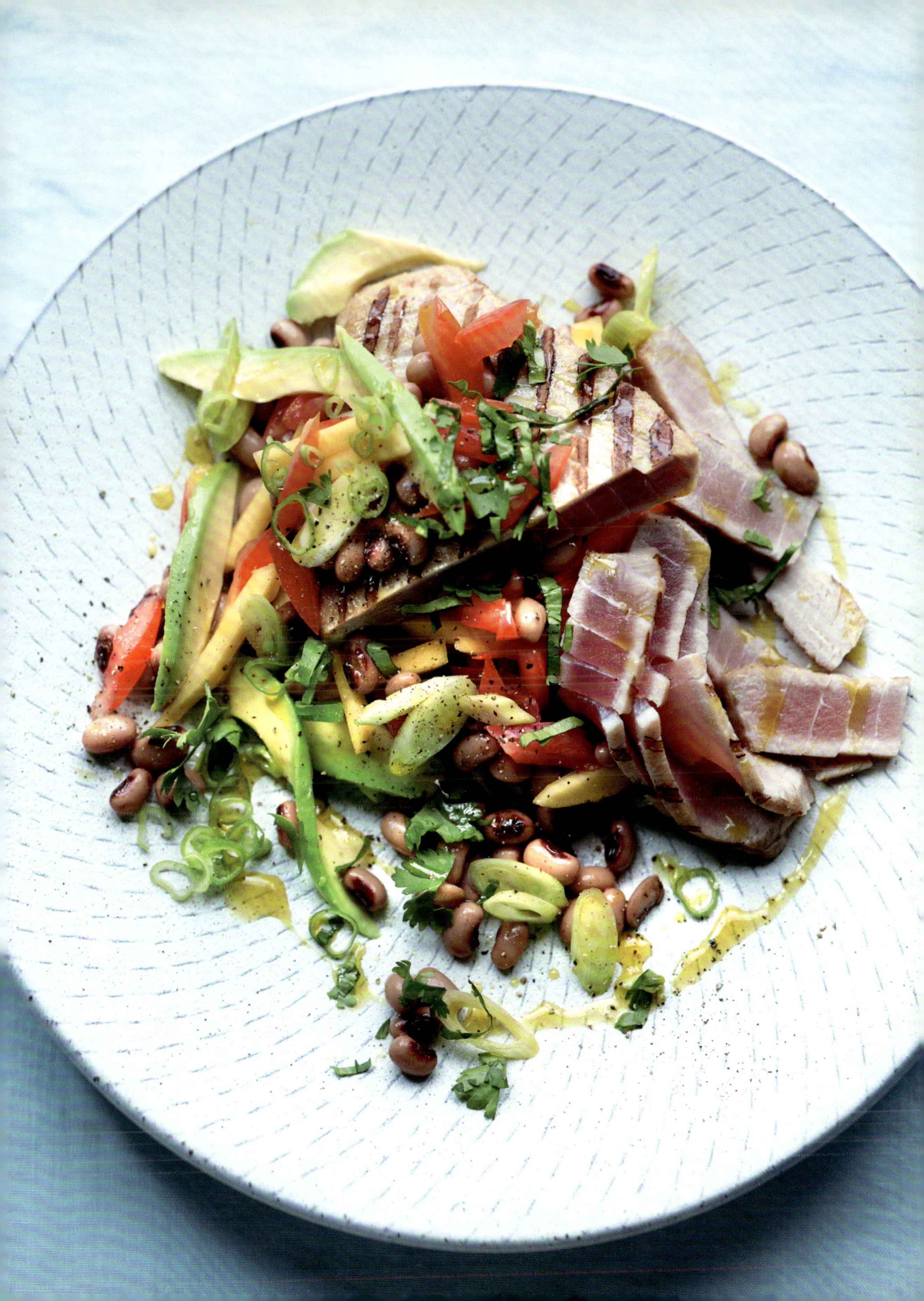

SERVES 2

MAKE AHEAD

GOOD TO FREEZE

(only the ratatouille, not the fish)

INGREDIENTS

- **1 tbsp coconut oil**
- **1 small red onion, roughly diced**
- **1 small courgette, cut into 1cm pieces**
- **1 small aubergine, cut into 1cm pieces**
- **1 sprig of thyme**
- **1 tbsp tomato puree**
- **2 tsp balsamic vinegar**
- **2 x 250g skinless salmon fillets**

QUICK POACHED SALMON WITH SPEEDY RAT-A-TAT-A-TOUILLE

Ratatouille doesn't have to take ages! Just make sure you chop all the vegetables to roughly the same, small size, so they cook quickly and evenly.

METHOD

Bring a large saucepan of water to the boil, ready to poach the salmon.

Meanwhile, melt the coconut oil in a large saucepan over a medium to high heat. Add the onion, courgette and aubergine and stir-fry for about 4 minutes or until they are just starting to soften and colour.

Drop in the thyme and stir for another minute, then squeeze in the tomato puree and mix to coat the vegetables. Keep frying, stirring continuously, for about 45 seconds before pouring in the balsamic vinegar and 100ml of water. Bring to the boil, then reduce to a simmer and let the ratatouille bubble away for about 10 minutes, or just until the vegetables are soft. If it seems to be getting too thick, add another 50ml or so of water.

While the veggies are simmering away, slide the salmon fillets into the boiling water. Bring back to a simmer, then cook the fish for 10 minutes, or until just cooked through.

Using a slotted spoon, carefully lift the fish out of the water and drain well. Serve up your yummy ratatouille topped with the juicy salmon.

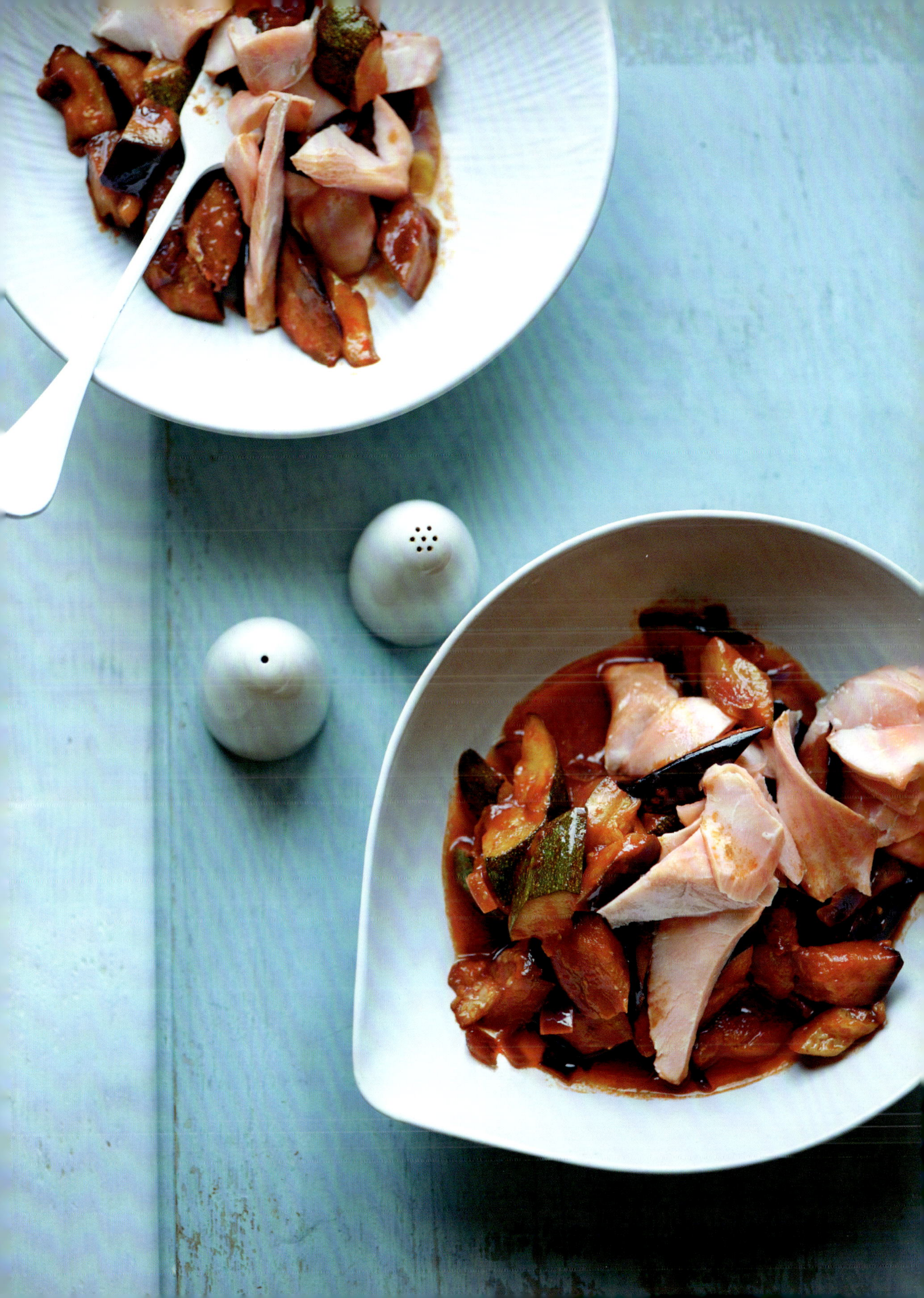

TURKEY MINCE LETTUCE BOATS

SERVES 2 (makes about 12 boats)

Spicy, fiery and packed with flavour, these little boats work as well for a dinner party as they do for a quick lunch. If you're bored of turkey mince, try making these with beef mince or prawns instead.

MAKE AHEAD

INGREDIENTS

- 1 tbsp coconut oil
- 500g turkey mince
- 5 spring onions, finely sliced
- 2 cloves garlic, finely chopped
- 1 red chilli, finely sliced – remove the seeds if you don't like it hot
- 1 tbsp fish sauce
- juice of 1 lime
- small bunch of coriander, leaves only, roughly chopped
- 2 avocados, roughly chopped
- 2 tomatoes, roughly chopped
- 2–3 baby gem lettuces, leaves separated

METHOD

Heat the coconut oil in a large frying pan over a high heat. Add the turkey mince and fry for 2–3 minutes, breaking up the mince as you cook. Add the spring onions, garlic and chilli and stir-fry for another 2 minutes, by which time the turkey mince should be cooked through. Add the fish sauce, lime juice and coriander. Mix everything together well, then remove the pan from the heat.

Combine the avocados and tomatoes in a bowl.

Lay out the lettuce leaves like little boats on your serving plate, then spoon in the turkey mixture and top with the avocados and tomatoes. Now go to munchies town and enjoy.

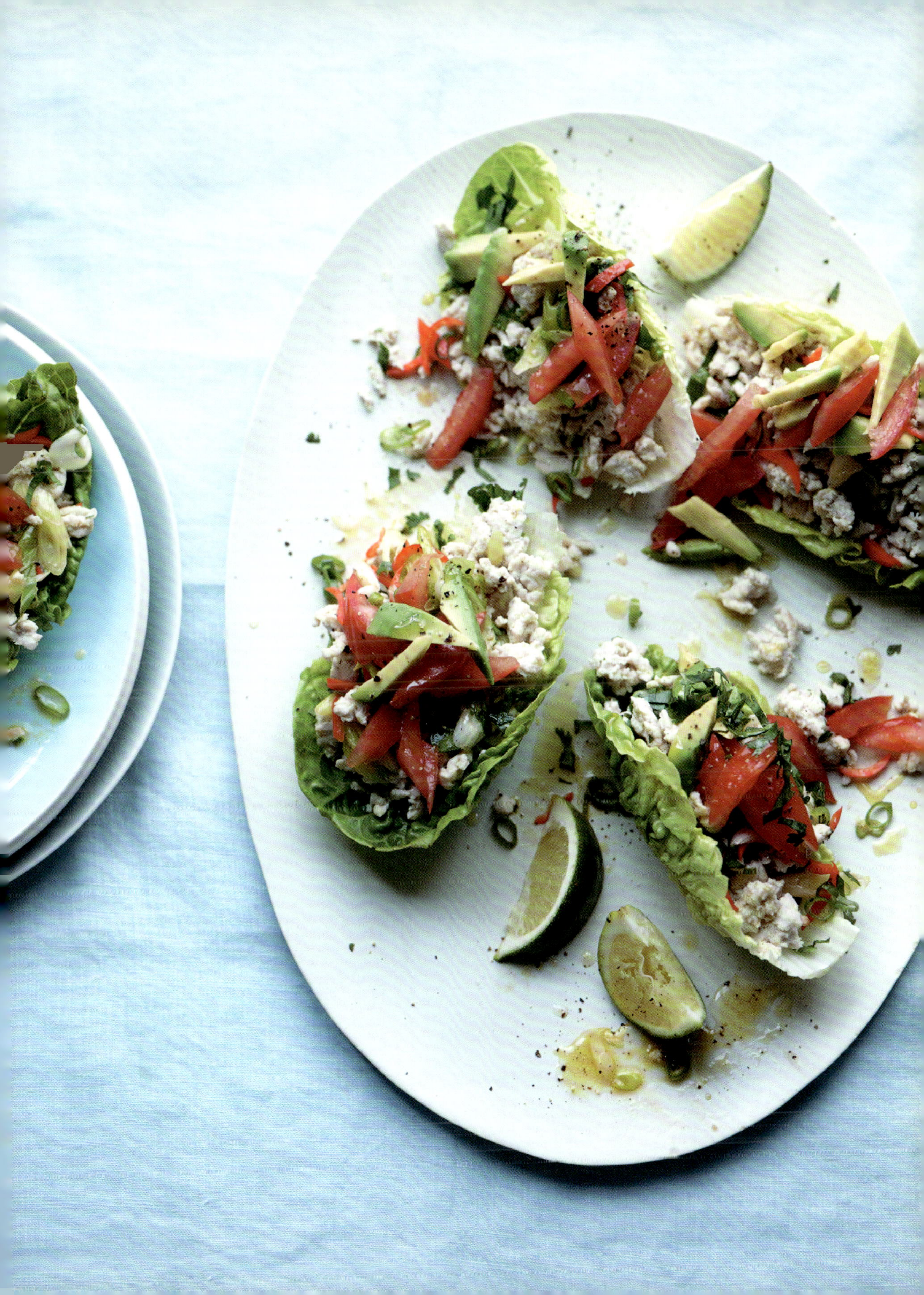

ITALIAN STALLION SAUSAGES

SERVES 2

MAKE AHEAD
GOOD TO FREEZE

INGREDIENTS

- 12 chipolata sausages
- 1 tbsp olive oil
- 1 tsp fennel seeds
- 2 shallots, roughly diced
- 1 clove garlic, roughly chopped
- 1 sprig of thyme
- 2 fennel bulbs, roughly diced
- 2 celery sticks, roughly diced
- 1 courgette, roughly diced
- 6 cherry tomatoes
- 1 tbsp tomato puree
- 250ml chicken stock
- ½ bunch of parsley, leaves only, roughly chopped

Oooh, if you love a bit of sausage, then this one's for you. It requires a few more ingredients than most of my Lean in 15 meals, but it's well worth the extra effort. This makes enough for two – or a meal for one, with the leftovers boxed up for the next day.

METHOD

Preheat your grill to maximum. Line up your chipolatas on the grill pan and cook for about 5 minutes on each side or until well browned and cooked through. Check by slicing into one of the sausages to make sure there are no raw pink bits left.

While the chipolatas are cooking, heat the oil in a large saucepan and fry the fennel seeds for about 20 seconds until they smell toasty. Add the shallots, garlic, thyme, fennel, celery and courgette and stir-fry for 2 minutes or until just starting to soften. Add the tomatoes and the tomato puree and keep stirring for another minute.

Pour in the chicken stock and bring to the boil, then reduce to a simmer. Slip the cooked chipolatas into the pan and let the whole lot bubble away for a minute. Stir through the parsley, then dish up.

★ Serve with a big portion of your favourite greens such as spinach, kale, broccoli, mange tout or green beans.

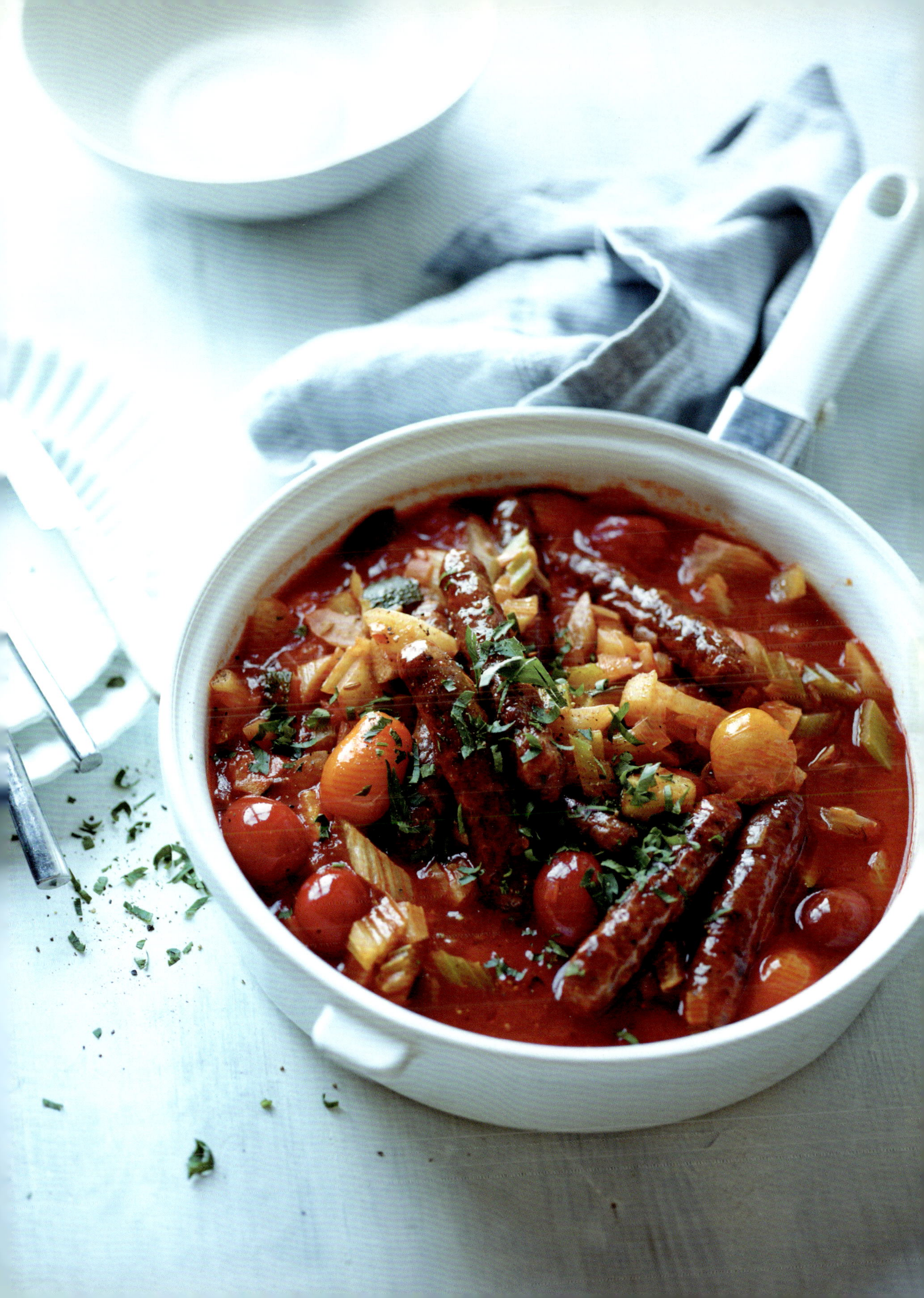

CREAMY STEAK AND SPINACH

SERVES 2

OMG – steak, wine and double cream? Am I dreaming? It feels naughty, but you'll love the taste of this one, and it's packed with healthy fats and protein.

INGREDIENTS

2 tbsp olive oil
2 x 250–300g sirloin steaks, trimmed of visible fat
salt and pepper
8 mushrooms, roughly chopped
splash of white wine
4 large handfuls of baby spinach leaves
75ml double cream

METHOD

Heat a frying pan over a high heat. Drizzle 1 tablespoon of the olive oil over the steaks, rubbing it into the flesh, and season all over with salt and pepper. Lay the steaks in the hot frying pan and cook for 3 minutes on each side. This will give you medium rare steak – if you prefer your meat medium or well done, increase the time until it's cooked to your liking. When you are happy with your steak, remove it from the frying pan and leave it to rest on a plate while you make your creamy side dish.

Wipe out the frying pan with a little kitchen roll, pour in the remaining olive oil and place over a medium to high heat. Add the mushrooms and cook, flipping them a couple of times, for 1–2 minutes or until lightly coloured. Season with salt and pepper and crank the heat up to maximum.

Pour in the white wine, and let it bubble away to almost nothing. Add the spinach and gently turn it in the pan until it is almost fully wilted. Pour in the double cream and let it bubble up. Check the seasoning and add more salt and pepper if needed.

Take a minute to look at what a delicious meal you've made, before wolfing it down!

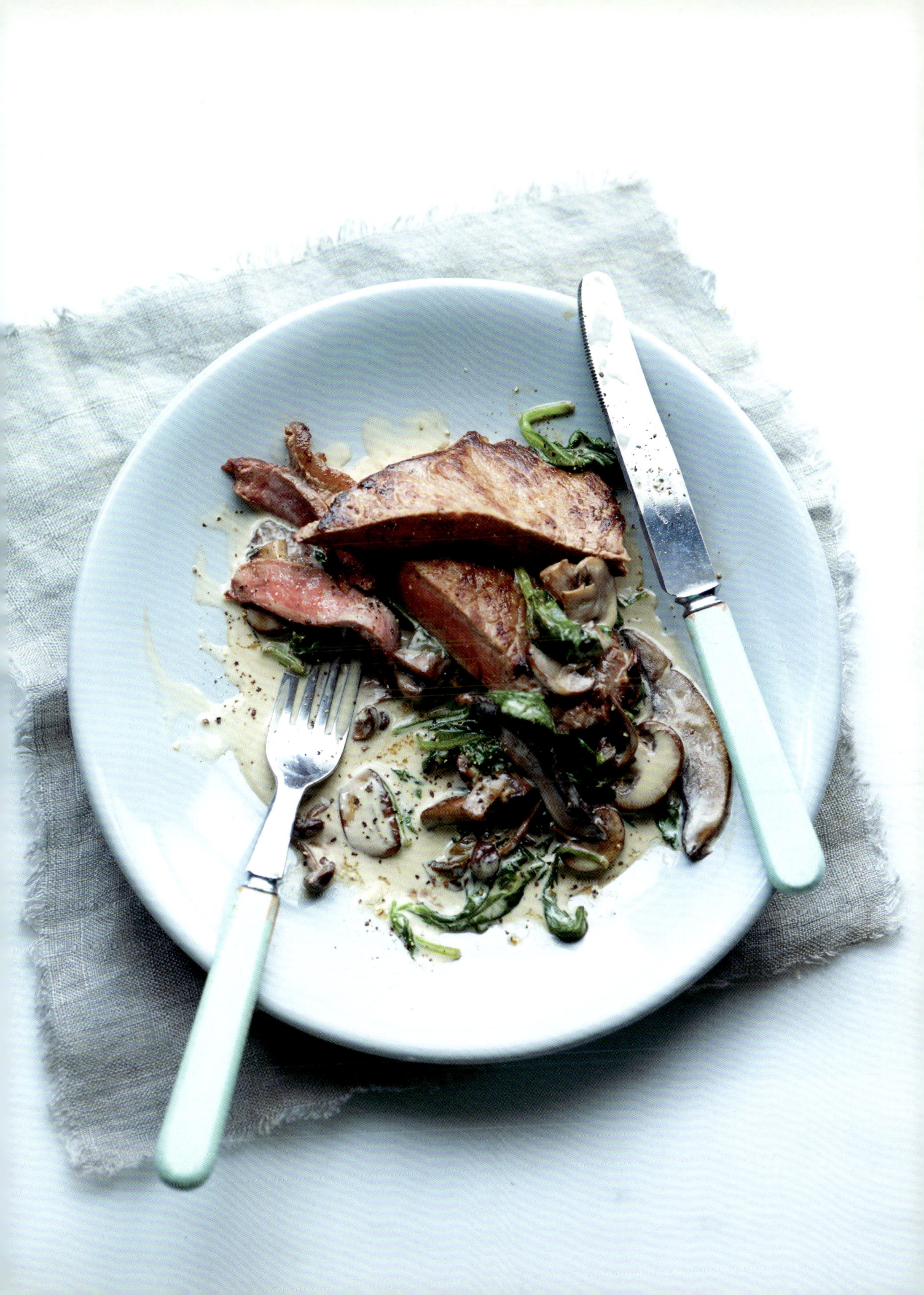

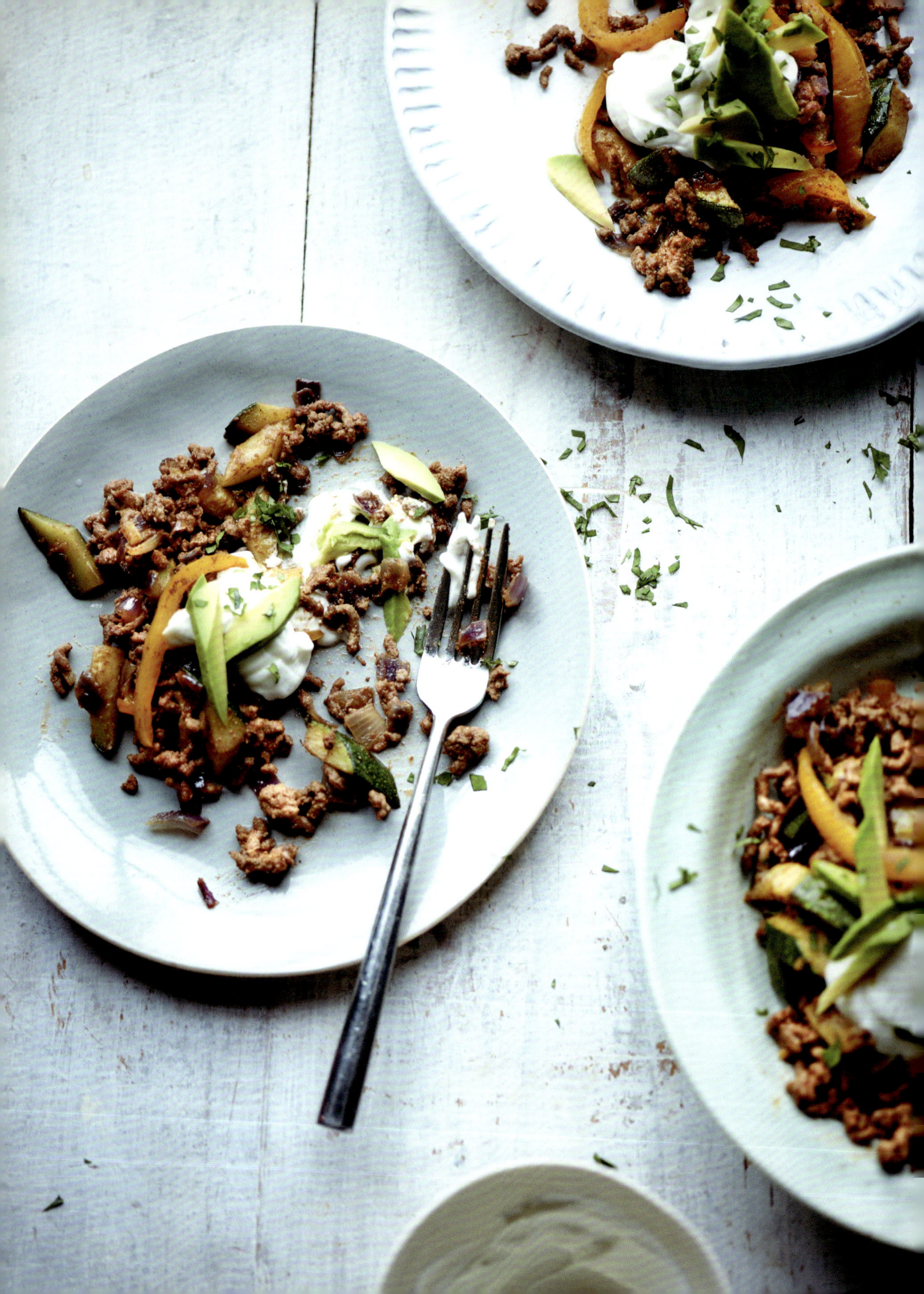

SERVES 1

CHILLI CON AVOCADO

This is a 'chuck everything in the pan' kinda dish: super-simple and tasty! It tastes great cold too, perfect for a packed lunch.

MAKE AHEAD

INGREDIENTS

½ tbsp coconut oil
1 small red onion, diced
1 green chilli, finely chopped – remove the seeds if you don't like it hot
1 red or yellow pepper, de-seeded and sliced
½ courgette, diced
300g reduced-fat (about 5%) beef mince
1 tsp smoked paprika
2 tsp ground cumin
salt and pepper
1 tbsp full-fat Greek yoghurt
½ avocado, sliced
½ bunch of coriander, leaves only, roughly chopped – optional

METHOD

Heat the coconut oil in a large frying pan over a high heat. Add the onion, chilli, pepper and courgette and stir-fry for 1–2 minutes or until the vegetables start to soften and colour.

Add the beef mince and stir to combine with the other ingredients, using your spoon to break up any large lumps as you go. Keep frying for about 3 minutes, by which time the mince should be fully cooked through.

Add the paprika and cumin, along with a generous pinch of salt and pepper, and cook for 30 seconds more.

Tip out your chilli onto a plate, then top with the yoghurt, avocado and coriander, if using, and serve.

GOAN FISH CURRY

SERVES 2

MAKE AHEAD
GOOD TO FREEZE

You don't need to go to India to enjoy a good curry. This recipe is surprisingly easy, but tastes incredible. If you're not fond of fish, you could always use 250g of skinless chicken breast fillet instead. This is a good meal to batch-cook and freeze when you're prepping like a boss . . .

INGREDIENTS

3 cloves garlic, roughly chopped
3cm ginger, roughly chopped
1 green chilli, roughly chopped – remove the seeds if you don't like it hot
2 tomatoes, roughly chopped
1 tbsp coconut oil
1 red onion, diced
1 tbsp garam masala
1 tbsp ground cumin
1 x 400ml tin of full-fat coconut milk
500g haddock fillet, skinned and cut into large chunks
juice of 1 lime
½ bunch of coriander, leaves only, roughly chopped

METHOD

Blitz the garlic, ginger, chilli and tomatoes in a food processor until smooth, then leave to one side.

Melt the oil in a wok or large frying pan over a medium to high heat. Throw in the onion and fry for 2 minutes, stirring regularly. Sprinkle in the garam masala and cumin and fry, stirring continuously, for 30 seconds. Pour in the blitzed ingredients and bring to the boil before pouring in the coconut milk. Return to the boil again, then let it simmer for 2 minutes.

Add the haddock pieces to the curry, and bring back to a simmer. Cook the fish for about 3 minutes, or until it is just cooked through.

Stir in the lime juice and coriander, then serve.

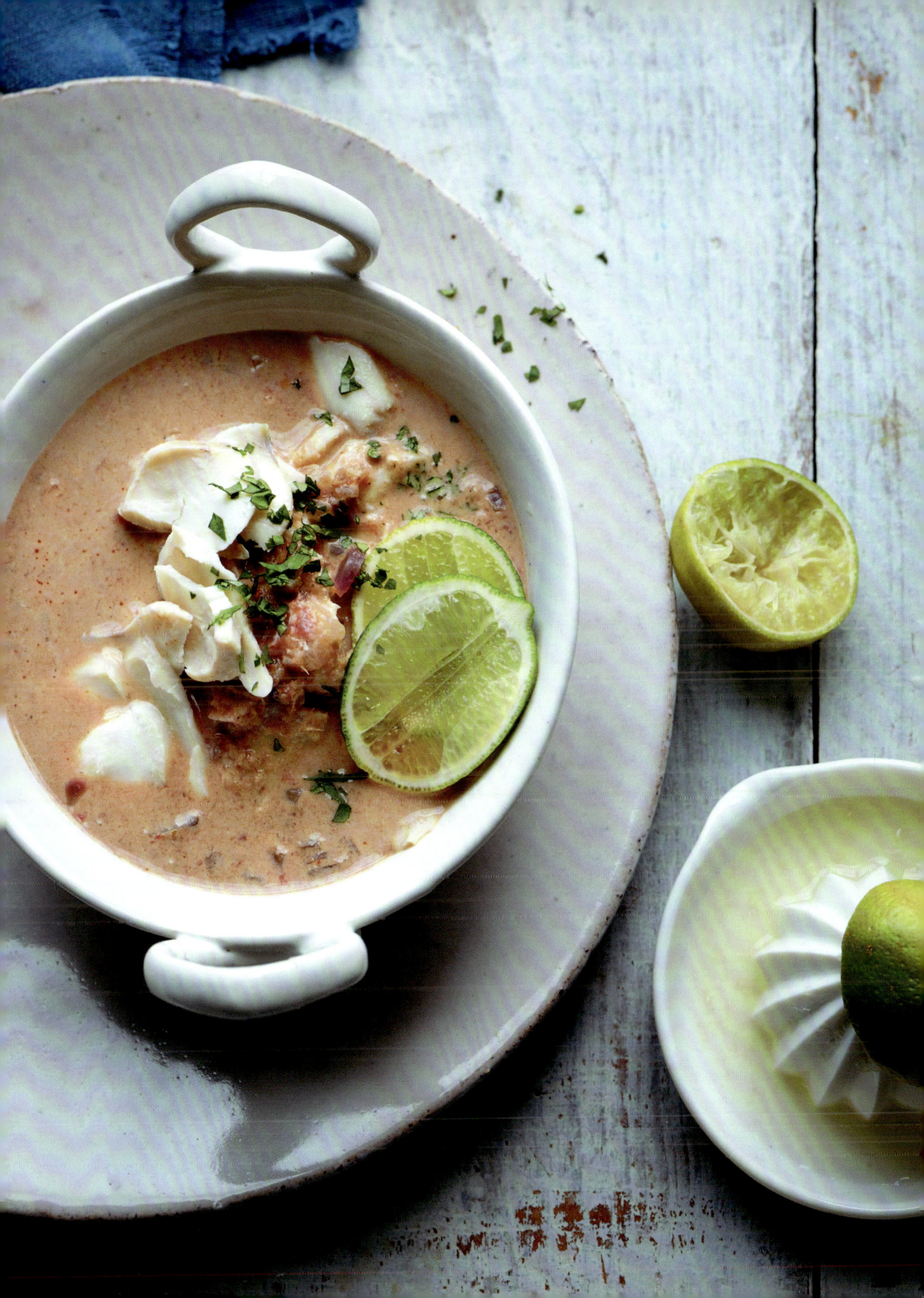

TOMATOES, EGGS AND CHORIZO

SERVES 1

If you love chorizo, this is perfect for you. Frying the chorizo with the tomatoes brings out all of the delicious flavour, and the eggs provide a dose of healthy fats.

INGREDIENTS

- ½ tbsp olive oil
- 75g chorizo (the cured type, not the softer cooking chorizo), chopped
- pinch of chilli flakes
- 2 spring onions, finely sliced
- 1 x 400g tin of chopped tomatoes
- 2 eggs
- 2 tbsp finely grated parmesan
- sprinkling of chopped parsley, if you're feeling fancy

METHOD

Heat the oil in a small frying pan. Add the chorizo, chilli flakes and spring onions and fry for about 2 minutes, stirring regularly.

Pour in the tomatoes and bring to the boil, then simmer for 1 minute. Reduce the heat to medium to low and use the back of a spoon to fashion two dips in the tomatoes as best you can. Crack an egg into each dip, sprinkle the parmesan over the eggs and place a lid on top (if you don't have a lid for your pan, a big dinner plate or a sheet of foil should work). Simmer for about 5–6 minutes or until the whites are cooked, but the yolks are still runny.

Sprinkle with chopped parsley, if you like, then gobble it up straight from the pan.

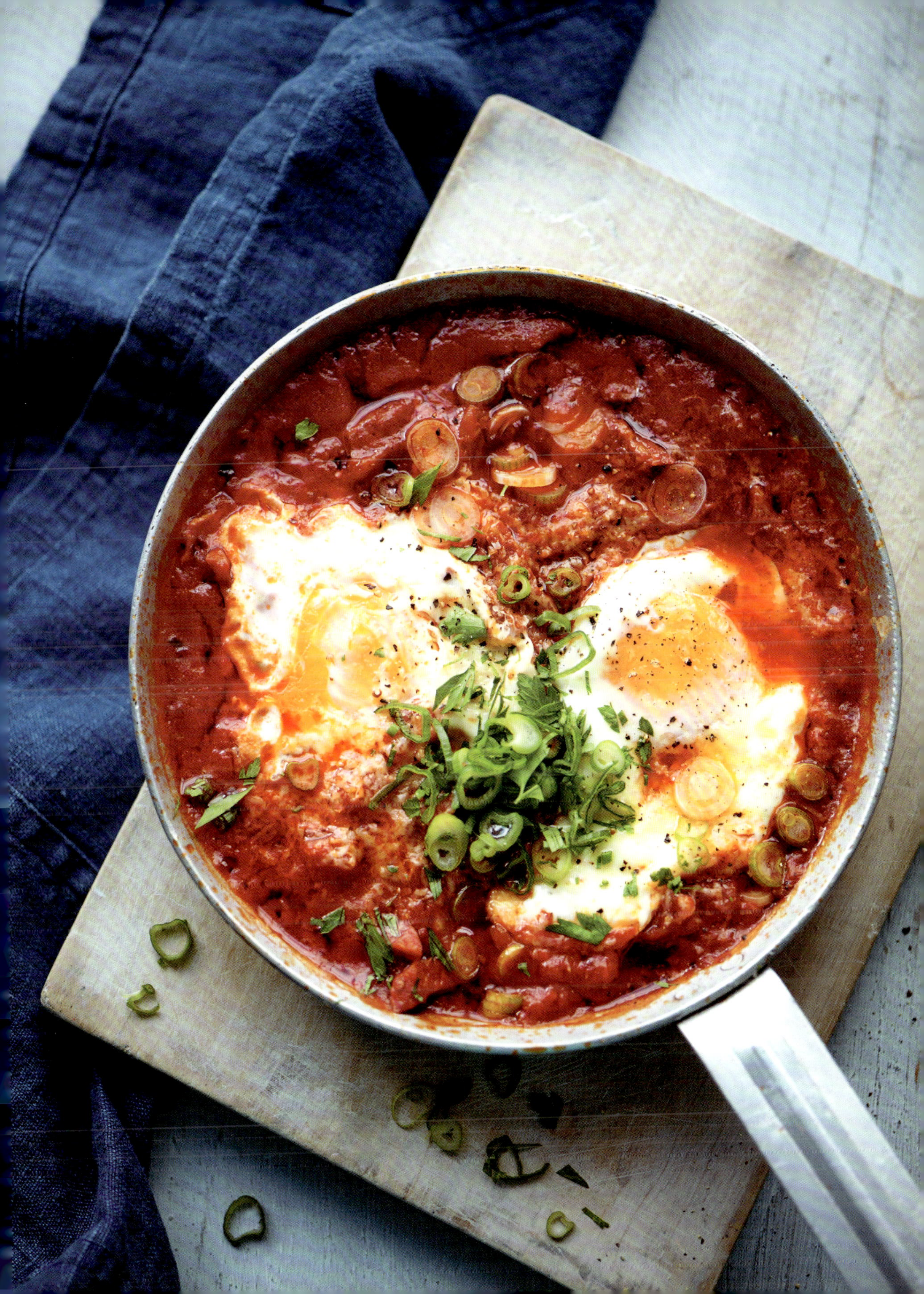

PRAWN AND BEANSPROUT OMELETTE

SERVES 1

This is my version of Egg Foo Yung, and it's a really quick breakfast option. Feel free to add other vegetables to the mix too.

INGREDIENTS

3 eggs
2 tsp light soy sauce
2 tsp toasted sesame oil
pepper
1 tbsp groundnut oil
200g cooked prawns
30g beansprouts
½ red chilli, finely sliced – remove the seeds if you don't like it hot
20g cashew nuts, roughly chopped
few leaves of coriander – optional

METHOD

Crack the eggs into a bowl and add the soy sauce and sesame oil, along with a grinding of black pepper. Beat together thoroughly.

Pour the groundnut oil into a small (about 15cm) non-stick frying pan over a high heat. When the oil is hot, pour the beaten egg mixture into the pan and use a wooden or plastic spoon to move the egg around as it cooks, a little like making scrambled eggs. When there is more firm egg than loose, turn the heat down to medium.

Lay the prawns on top of the omelette, followed by the beansprouts. Fold the omelette in half over the filling and let everything warm through for 30 seconds.

Gently tip your omelette onto a plate and top with the red chilli, cashew nuts and coriander leaves, if using.

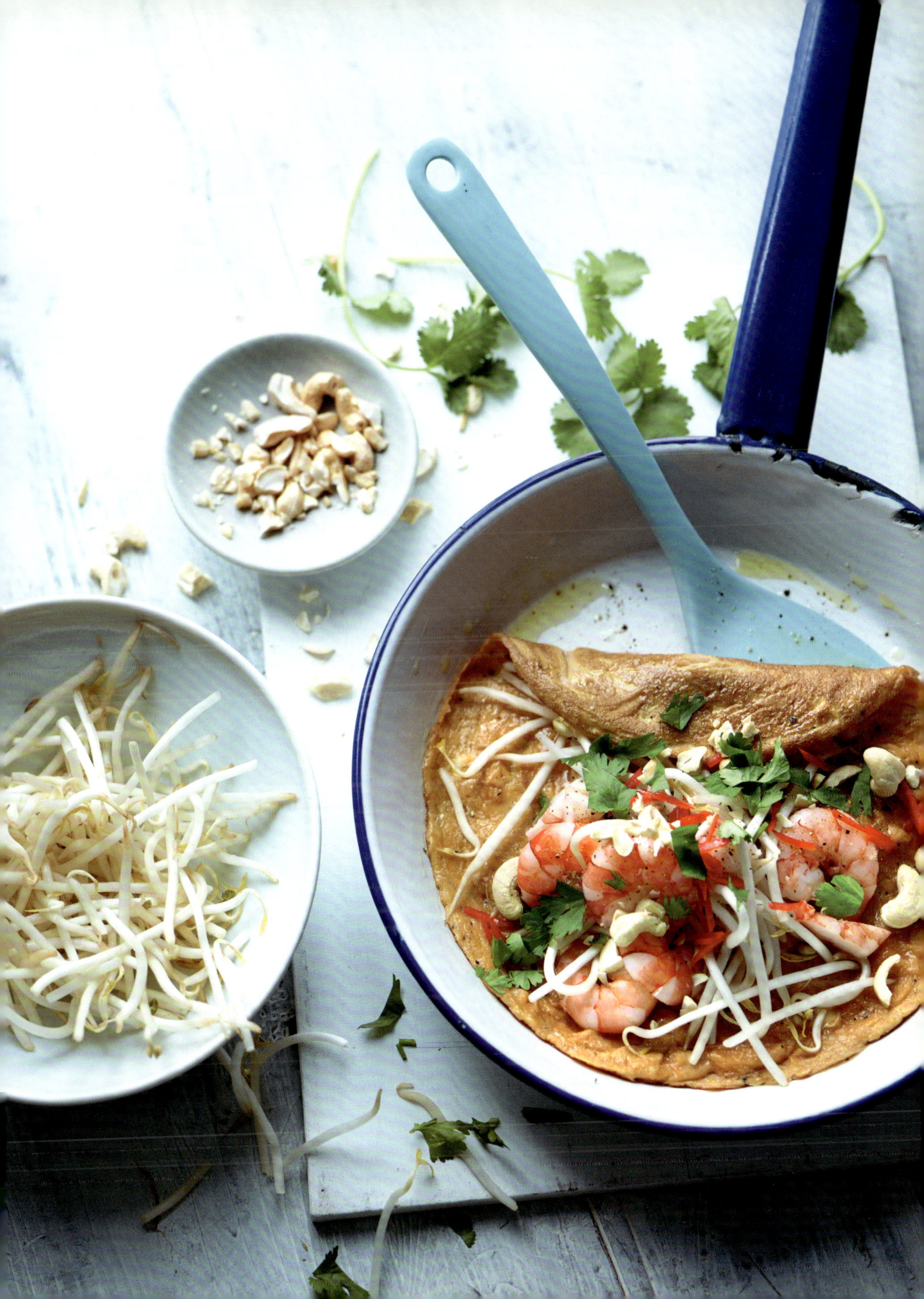

POACHED SALMON WITH BACON

SERVES 2

Mmm, bacon and salmon. Yes, please! This dish is a real winner on flavour, and it's full of those essential omega-3 fatty acids that will help to keep you lean.

MAKE AHEAD

INGREDIENTS

- 2 x 250g skinless salmon fillets
- ½ tbsp olive oil
- 2 rashers of thick smoked back bacon, trimmed of visible fat and sliced into 1cm strips
- 1 courgette, cut into half moons
- 200g midget trees (tender-stem broccoli), any bigger stalks sliced in half lengthways
- 8 cherry tomatoes
- 2 handfuls of baby spinach leaves
- salt and pepper
- 40g pine nuts
- finely grated parmesan, to serve

METHOD

Bring a large saucepan of water to the boil. Carefully slide the salmon fillets into the water and reduce the heat to just simmering. Poach the fish for 10 minutes or until just cooked through. Using a slotted spoon, carefully lift the fish out of the water and drain well.

While the fish is cooking, heat the oil in a large frying pan over a medium to high heat. When the oil is hot, fry the bacon for 1 minute, then add the courgette and midget trees and fry for another minute. Throw in the cherry tomatoes and cook for a further minute or until the tomatoes start to burst open and leak some of their delicious juices. Add the spinach and let it wilt down, then season with a little salt and a generous amount of pepper.

Divide the bacon and vegetable mixture between two plates, top with the poached salmon and finish with a scattering of pine nuts. Serve with a little finely grated parmesan.

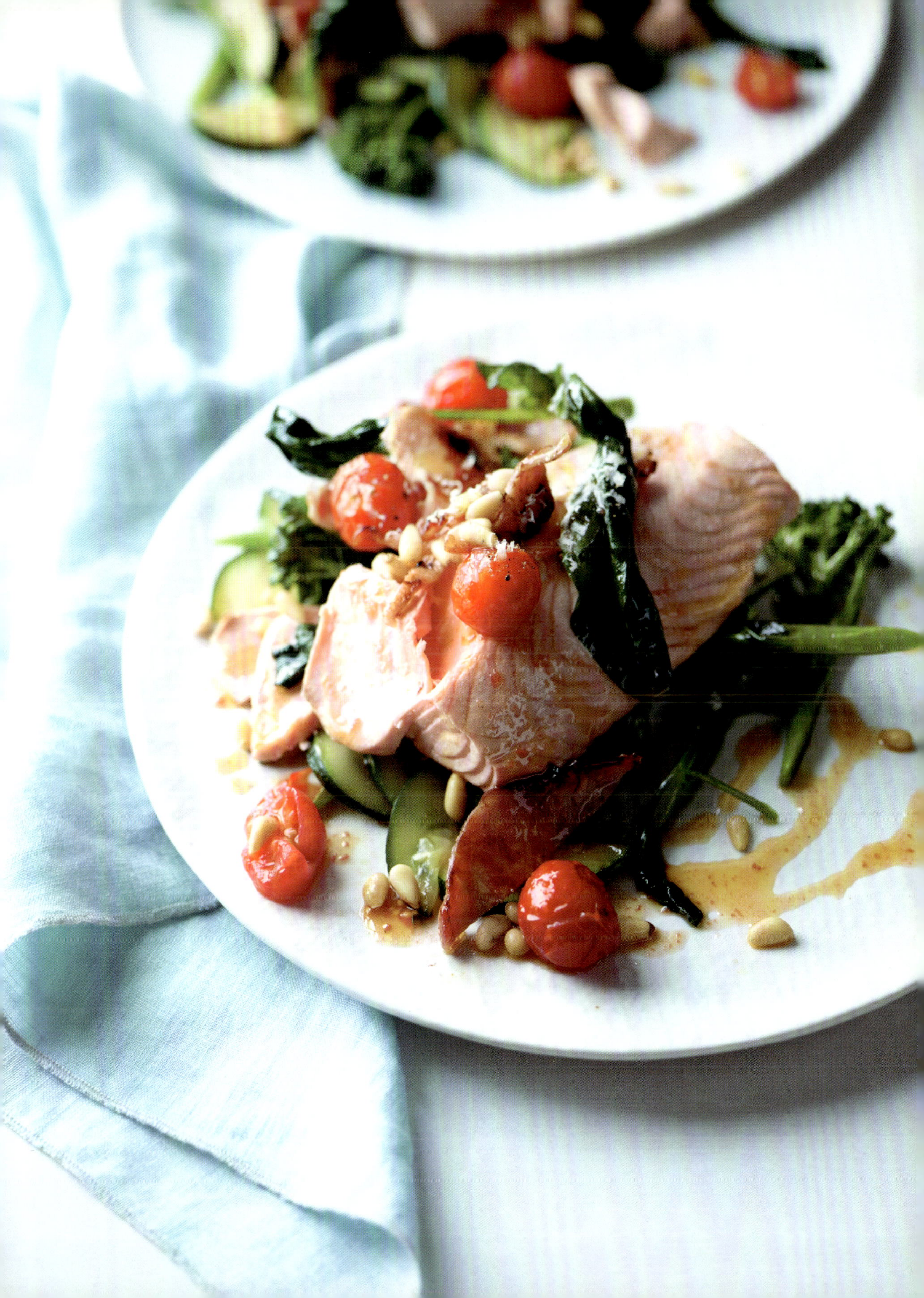

SEA BASS WITH SPICED CAULIFLOWER, PEAS AND PANEER

SERVES 2

The Indian fresh cheese known as paneer is very similar to halloumi, and it goes perfectly with the sea bass and cauliflower in this dish. Feel free to use halloumi if you can't find paneer. Garam masala is a store cupboard essential and brings a big boost of flavour to almost anything!

INGREDIENTS

- 1 small cauliflower, broken into florets
- 1 tbsp coconut oil
- 1 red onion, diced
- 2cm ginger, finely chopped
- 150g paneer, roughly diced into 2cm cubes
- 1 tbsp garam masala
- 125g frozen peas
- 2 handfuls of baby spinach leaves
- ½ bunch of coriander, leaves only, roughly chopped
- 4 x 120g fillets of sea bass, skin on, but scaled
- salt and pepper
- juice of 1 lime

METHOD

Bring a large saucepan of water to the boil, then drop in the cauliflower florets and cook for 3 minutes. Drain in a sieve or colander, then rinse under cold running water. Leave the florets cooling in the sieve or colander.

In a large frying pan or wok, heat half the coconut oil over a medium to high heat. Add the onion and stir-fry for 2 minutes or until just starting to soften, then add the ginger and stir-fry for a further minute.

Add the paneer, garam masala and peas and keep stir-frying for 1–2 minutes, or until the peas have defrosted and are warmed through. If the garam masala seems to be catching on the bottom of the pan and burning, just add a drizzle of water. Chuck in the spinach, cauliflower and coriander and stir until the spinach has wilted.

In a separate frying pan, heat the rest of the coconut oil over a medium to high heat. Season the fish fillets with salt and pepper and, when the oil is hot, lay the fish in the pan, skin side down. Fry without turning for 1–2 minutes until the skin is crisp, then flip the fish over and cook for a final minute.

Divide the paneer and vegetables between two plates and top with the sea bass. Finish with a squeeze of lime juice.

CODDLED EGGS WITH SPINACH AND BACON

SERVES 1

Coddled eggs are basically steamed, creamy eggs. I love their texture, but if you would rather have poached or scrambled eggs, then go for it.

INGREDIENTS

- large knob of butter
- 2 large eggs
- ½ tbsp olive oil
- 4 rashers of smoked back bacon, trimmed of visible fat and sliced into 1cm thick strips
- 2 large handfuls of baby spinach leaves
- salt and pepper
- 2 tbsp pine nuts

METHOD

Bring a large saucepan of water to the boil and set a steamer basket on top.

Drop a chunk of butter into two ramekin dishes, then crack an egg into each one. When the water is boiling and there is a good amount of steam running through the steamer, carefully place the ramekins into the basket. Cover and steam the eggs for 6–10 minutes or until the whites are firm, but the yolks are still runny.

Meanwhile, heat the olive oil in a large frying pan over a medium to high heat. Add the bacon and fry for 1–2 minutes or until crisp. Stir in the spinach and cook until it has wilted, then season with salt and pepper.

Serve up the coddled eggs with the bacon and spinach, topped with a sprinkling of pine nuts.

SALMON WITH CAPERS AND CAPRESE SALAD

SERVES 2

Close your eyes when you eat this and you could be in Italy: Caprese salad, capers and fresh basil. What a combo!

MAKE AHEAD

INGREDIENTS

- 4 tbsp light olive oil
- 2 x 250g skinless salmon fillets
- 1 tsp Dijon mustard
- juice of ½ lemon
- 2 tsp capers
- 1 avocado, roughly diced
- 2 ripe tomatoes, roughly chopped
- 1 ball of mozzarella, torn into pieces
- small handful of basil leaves
- 50g walnuts, roughly chopped

METHOD

Heat 1 tablespoon of the olive oil in a frying pan over a medium to high heat. Add the salmon fillets and fry for 1–2 minutes on each side, by which time the fish should be lightly coloured. Using a spatula, break the fish into large chunks and fry for a further 2–3 minutes or until the fish is just cooked through. Remove the pan from the heat and transfer the salmon to a plate.

Mix together the mustard, lemon juice, capers and the remaining olive oil to make a dressing.

Arrange the avocado, tomato and mozzarella over two plates. Top with the salmon chunks, scatter with the basil leaves and walnuts, and finally spoon over the dressing.

★ TOP TIP

Buy herb plants, sit them in a window box or on a windowsill and you'll have free herbs forever.

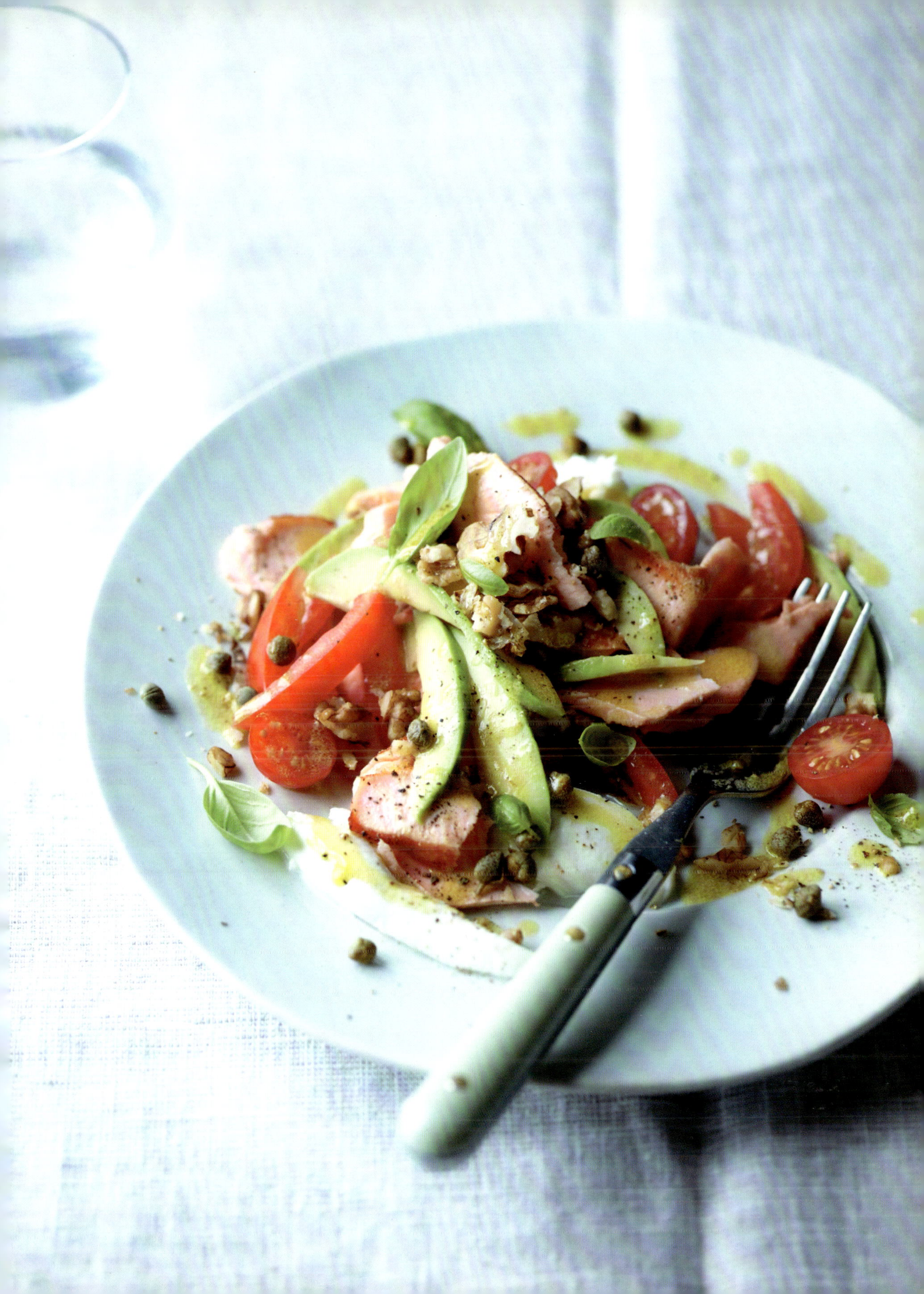

TERIYAKI SALMON WITH COURGETTE NOODLES

SERVES 1

MAKE AHEAD

INGREDIENTS

- ½ tbsp coconut oil
- 1 x 240g skinless salmon fillet
- 2 spring onions, finely sliced
- 2cm ginger, finely chopped
- 2 tbsp light soy sauce
- 1 tbsp honey
- ½ tbsp rice wine vinegar
- 4 cherry tomatoes, cut in half
- 1 large courgette, spiralized or sliced to make long noodle-like strands
- 2 tsp sesame oil

If you don't have a spiralizer, make the courgette noodles by using a peeler to create long thin ribbons of courgette, which you can then stack up and slice with a knife into noodle-like strips.

METHOD

Heat half of the coconut oil in a frying pan over a medium to high heat. When the oil is melted and hot, slide in the salmon and fry for 2–3 minutes on each side or until lightly browned and almost cooked through.

Meanwhile, mix together the spring onions, ginger, soy sauce, honey and vinegar to make a teriyaki sauce. Pour this into the pan with the salmon and let it bubble up, then remove the pan from the heat.

In another frying pan, heat the remaining coconut oil over a high heat. Tumble in the tomatoes and stir-fry for 1 minute. Gently add the courgette noodles and lightly toss for 1 minute just to warm through.

Plate up the noodles and tomatoes, then top with the teriyaki salmon. Finish with a little drizzle of sesame oil.

SERVES 2

MAKE AHEAD
(but reheat in the oven, not in the microwave)
GOOD TO FREEZE

INGREDIENTS

- 50g rolled oats
- 50g ground almonds
- 3 tsp smoked paprika
- salt and pepper
- 1 egg
- 2 x 220g skinless chicken breast fillets
- 2 tbsp plain flour
- 1 tbsp coconut oil
- ½ cucumber, roughly chopped into 2cm pieces
- 1 large tomato, roughly chopped
- 1 avocado, roughly chopped
- 1 tbsp olive oil
- squeeze of lemon juice

MY OATY CHICKEN

Feeling stressed out after a long day at work? Cook this meal and you can take it out on your chicken, as you get to give it a good bash with a rolling pin or your fists to make it cook more quickly. Oh, and did I mention it's covered in an oaty, nutty crispy coating that tastes out of this world when you fry it in coconut oil?

METHOD

In a shallow dish, mix together the rolled oats, ground almonds, smoked paprika and a generous pinch of salt and pepper. Crack the egg into another shallow bowl and whisk.

Lay a large sheet of cling film on your chopping board and place the chicken breasts on it, allowing room for them to spread, then place another sheet of cling film on top. Using a rolling pin, meat hammer or other blunt instrument, bash the breasts until they are half their original thickness and flattened out. Remove the chicken breasts from the cling film and dust all over with the flour, shaking them lightly to remove any excess, then dip into the beaten egg, again shaking off any excess. Finally, dunk the chicken breasts into the oat and almond mixture, pressing it on to cover both sides as well as you can.

Heat the coconut oil in a large non-stick frying pan over a medium heat. Carefully lay the chicken breasts into the oil and fry for about 4 minutes on each side or until the chicken is cooked through. Check by cutting into the thickest part to make sure the meat is white, with no signs of pink. Transfer the chicken to paper towels to drain off any excess oil.

Mix together the cucumber, tomato, avocado, olive oil and lemon juice to make a quick salad, then serve alongside the oaty chicken.

MUSSELS IN COCONUT MILK

SERVES 2

If you've never tried mussels cooked in coconut milk, you're in for a treat. They make a nice change from fish or prawns, and they taste great.

INGREDIENTS

- 1 tbsp coconut oil
- 2 star anise
- 6 spring onions, finely sliced
- 2 cloves garlic, finely chopped
- 1 lemongrass stalk, bruised with the back of a knife
- 1 red chilli, roughly chopped – remove the seeds if you don't like it hot
- 1 x 400ml tin of full-fat coconut milk
- 2kg mussels, shells scrubbed and beards removed
- 2 tbsp fish sauce
- small bunch of coriander, leaves only, roughly chopped
- 2 limes

METHOD

Heat the coconut oil in a very large pan or wok for which you have a lid (or you can improvise with a large dinner plate or a sheet of foil). When the oil has melted, add the star anise, spring onions, garlic, lemongrass and chilli and stir-fry for 1 minute or until the spring onions and garlic are starting to soften – by now the smell should be getting your appetite going too!

Pour in the coconut milk and bring to the boil, then reduce the heat and simmer for about 3 minutes to reduce the liquid a little. Check your mussels at this point: if there are any that are open and do not clamp shut when tapped, throw them away. Tumble the mussels into the coconut milk and give them a stir, then cover and cook for 3–4 minutes, shaking the pan every now and then. The mussels are cooked when their shells are fully open – be careful not to overcook, as that's how they become chewy. Discard any mussels that don't open up.

Remove the pan from the heat and stir in the fish sauce, half of the chopped coriander and the juice of one of the limes. Divide the mussels between two bowls and garnish with the rest of the coriander. Cut the other lime in half and serve on the side of the bowl, for squeezing.

★ Serve with a big portion of your favourite greens such as spinach, kale, broccoli, mange tout or green beans.

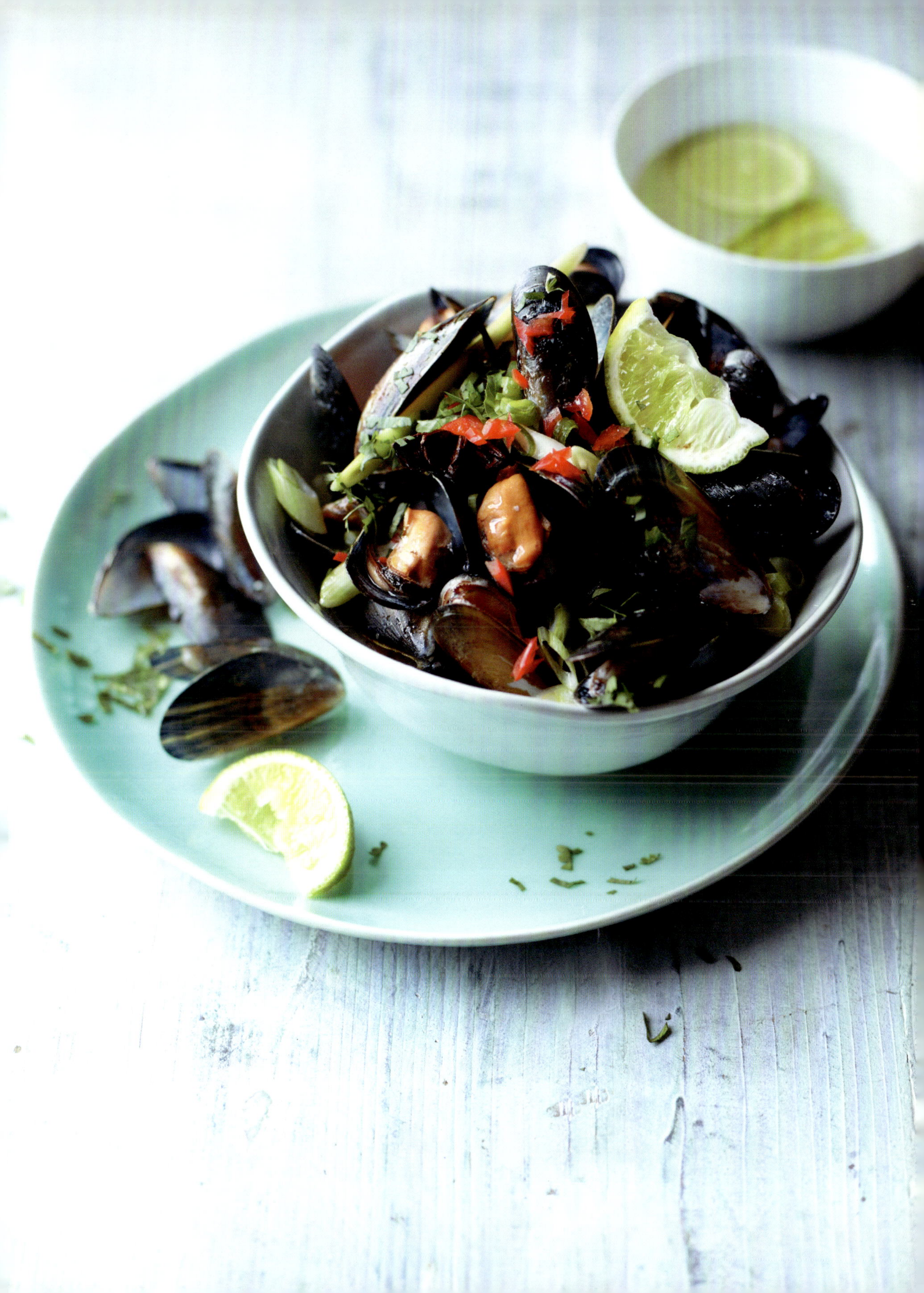

STEAK WITH SPICY CHORIZO, TOMATOES AND KALE

SERVES 2

Ooh, steak and chorizo in one dish? Count me in! This is a real meat lover's dish. If you're not a fan of kale, you could always use spinach, but be sure to get your greens in.

INGREDIENTS

2 tbsp olive oil
2 x 240g sirloin steaks, trimmed of visible fat
salt and pepper
75g cured chorizo, diced
200g kale, thick stalks removed
8 cherry tomatoes, cut in half
1 tbsp sherry vinegar, or balsamic or red wine vinegar

METHOD

Bring a large saucepan of water to the boil, and place a frying pan over a high heat.

Rub the olive oil all over the steaks and season generously with salt and pepper. When the pan is very hot, carefully lay the steaks in it and fry for 2 minutes before flipping and frying for another 2 minutes. Transfer the steak to a plate and leave to rest.

Meanwhile, throw the chorizo into the same frying pan, turn the heat down to low and cook for about 2 minutes. At the same time, drop the kale into the boiling water and simmer for 1 minute, then drain in a sieve or colander.

Crank up the heat under the chorizo to maximum, then add the tomatoes to the pan and stir-fry for 1 minute. Pour in the vinegar and let it bubble away to almost nothing. Add the kale and toss to combine everything thoroughly.

Remove from the heat and season to taste with salt and pepper. Place a steak on each plate and top with the delicious stir-fry.

CLASSIC SMOKED SALMON AND SCRAMBLED EGGS

SERVES 2

The king of healthy breakfasts is a true Lean in 15 dish! If you're always in a rush in the morning, this one's for you. Scrambling the eggs on a low heat with butter gives them a seriously creamy texture.

INGREDIENTS

6 eggs
20g butter, roughly chopped
pepper
6 slices smoked salmon, cut into 1cm thick strips
small bunch of chives, finely sliced
handful of baby spinach leaves, to serve

METHOD

Bring a saucepan of water to the boil.

Crack the eggs into a large heatproof bowl and add the butter, along with a good grinding of pepper. Whisk the eggs together, then sit the bowl over the pan of boiling water and immediately reduce the heat to a simmer. Cook the eggs for about 10 minutes, stirring regularly. As the eggs begin to scramble, add the smoked salmon and the chives, and keep cooking the eggs until they reach your preferred consistency – the longer you cook them, the firmer they'll get.

Serve up these luxurious eggs with a big handful of spinach and a final grinding of black pepper.

SEA BASS WITH BRAZIL NUTS, KALE AND POMEGRANATE

SERVES 1

MAKE AHEAD

INGREDIENTS

- 2 tbsp olive oil
- 2 x 120g sea bass fillets, skin on
- salt and pepper
- 75g kale, thick stalks removed
- 4 midget trees (tender-stem broccoli), any bigger stalks sliced in half lengthways
- 2 tbsp pomegranate seeds
- 25g brazil nuts, chopped
- 1 red chilli, finely sliced – remove the seeds if you don't like it hot

Sea bass with nuts and pomegranate – such a great combination of flavours and packed with goodness. This is a dish to impress your friends at a dinner party!

METHOD

Bring a saucepan of water to the boil.

Meanwhile, heat half of the olive oil in a frying pan over a medium to high heat. Season the sea bass with salt and pepper and, when the oil is hot, carefully lay the fish in the pan, skin side down. Cook, without turning, for 2–3 minutes, then carefully flip it over. Remove the pan from the heat and let the fish finish cooking in the residual heat.

Drop the kale and midget trees into the boiling water and simmer for 2 minutes. Drain in a sieve or colander, then rinse under cold running water. Transfer the vegetables to a bowl and add the rest of the olive oil, along with the pomegranate seeds, brazil nuts and chilli. Gently toss everything together.

Pile the vegetables onto the plate, sit the fish on top, and tuck in.

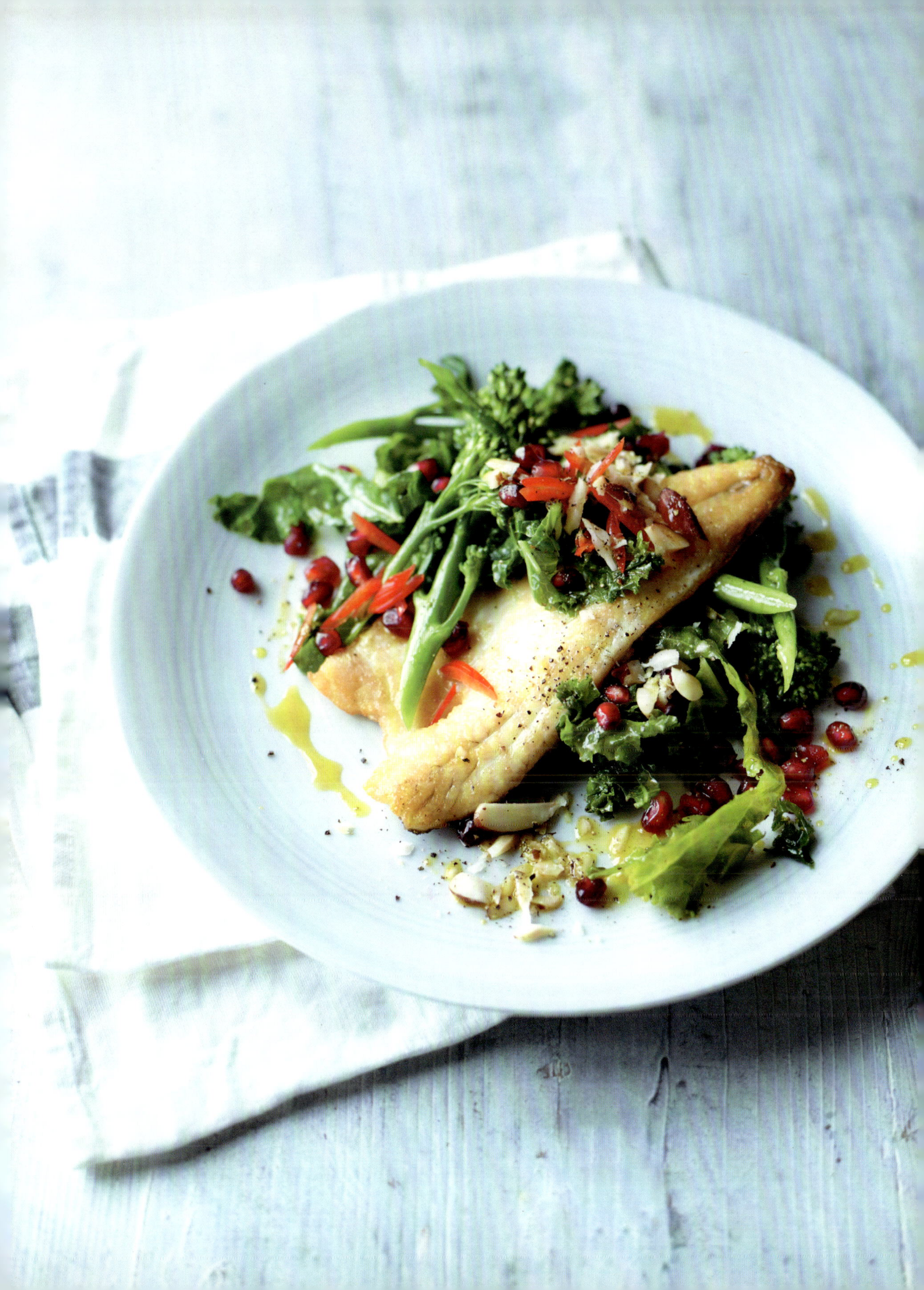

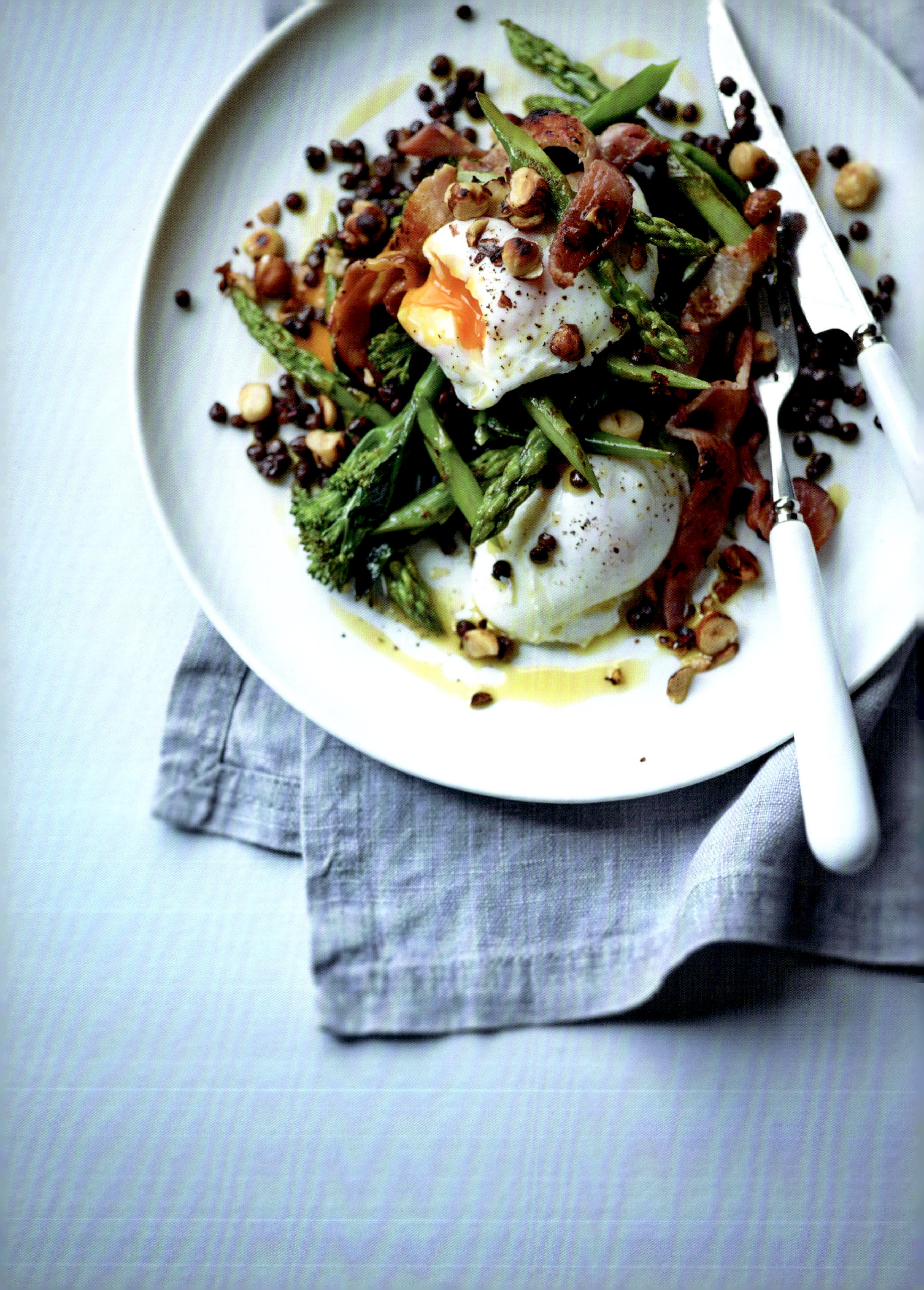

GRIDDLED MIDGET TREES AND SPEARS WITH EGGS

SERVES 2

What can I say? You know how obsessed I am with midget trees! Well, here's a breakfast idea I'm sure you'll love as much as I do.

INGREDIENTS

- 8 spears of asparagus, woody parts of stalks removed
- 8 midget trees (tender-stem broccoli)
- 2 rashers of smoked back bacon
- salt and pepper
- 150g pre-cooked puy lentils
- 4 eggs
- glug of olive oil
- splash of sherry vinegar
- 2 tbsp toasted and chopped hazelnuts

METHOD

Bring a large saucepan of water to the boil and place a griddle pan over a high heat. It's probably best to throw open a window too, as griddling always seems to set the smoke alarm off . . .

When the griddle pan is hot, place the spears, trees and bacon directly onto it, sprinkling the vegetables with a little salt and pepper. Cook for 3–4 minutes, turning regularly – you're after crispy bacon and lightly chargrilled vegetables.

Ping the lentils in the microwave according to the packet instructions.

Carefully crack your eggs into the hot water, reducing the heat until the water is just 'burping'. Cook the eggs for about 4 minutes for a runny yolk, then carefully lift them out with a slotted spoon and drain on paper towels.

Once the veg are all cooked, scoop them up and drop them into a large bowl. Remove the bacon and roughly chop, then add to the bowl too, along with the olive oil, sherry vinegar and lentils. Season to taste with salt and pepper and toss the whole lot together before piling onto plates. Top with the poached eggs and finish with the toasted hazelnuts.

DUCK, GREEN BEANS AND WALNUTS

SERVES 1

MAKE AHEAD

Oh, hello, healthy fats! Although this feels like a high-end bistro dish, it's ready in minutes. And as it's just as tasty eaten at room temperature, it works very well as a packed lunch too.

INGREDIENTS

1 tbsp olive oil
240g duck breast fillet, sliced into 2cm thick strips
salt and pepper
100g green beans
1 tbsp walnut oil
40g walnuts
2 tbsp sundried tomatoes

METHOD

Bring a large saucepan of water to the boil.

Heat the olive oil in a frying pan over a medium to high heat. Season the duck breast with salt and pepper. When the oil is hot, add the duck and fry, stirring occasionally, for about 3 minutes or until the duck is cooked through and lightly golden in places.

Meanwhile, drop the beans into the boiling water and simmer for 1 minute. Drain in a sieve or colander, then rinse under cold running water. Tip the beans into a bowl and add the walnut oil, walnuts and sundried tomatoes. Season generously with salt and pepper, then toss everything together.

Arrange the green beans and walnuts on a plate and top with the duck.

TURKEY MEATBALLS WITH FETA

SERVES 1

MAKE AHEAD
GOOD TO FREEZE

INGREDIENTS

½ tbsp coconut oil
½ red onion, diced
1 red or yellow pepper, de-seeded and thinly sliced
½ courgette, diced
300g ready-made turkey meatballs (available at most supermarkets)
1 x 400g tin of chopped tomatoes
20g feta, crumbled
½ bunch of parsley, leaves only, roughly chopped – optional

These meatballs went down a treat on Instagram, ranking as one of my most popular videos. The cheesy sauce also tastes great with beef meatballs. Feel free to throw in any extra veg you have left in the fridge too.

METHOD

Heat the coconut oil in a large frying pan over a medium to high heat. Add the onion, pepper and courgette, and stir-fry for 2 minutes until the vegetables begin to soften and wilt.

Increase the heat to maximum and roll the meatballs into the pan. Fry for 2–3 minutes, moving them frequently so they brown all over.

Pour in the chopped tomatoes and bring to the boil, then reduce the heat and simmer for 5 minutes, or until the meatballs are fully cooked through. To check, cut the largest one in half and make sure all the meat has turned from pink to white.

Remove the pan from the heat, crumble over the feta and sprinkle with parsley, if using.

★ TOP TIP

If you can't find ready-made turkey meatballs in your supermarket, simply buy turkey mince and season it with a generous amount of salt and pepper. Create some extra flavour by adding in a pinch of dried oregano, parsley or Cajun spice. Knead for a minute and then form into golfball-sized meatballs.

LAMB KOFTAS WITH GREEK SALAD

SERVES 2

MAKE AHEAD
GOOD TO FREEZE
(the koftas, not the salad!)

INGREDIENTS

350g lean lamb mince
2 tsp ground cinnamon
2 tsp ground cumin
4 spring onions, finely sliced
2 cloves garlic, finely chopped
salt and pepper
½ cucumber, roughly chopped into big chunks
1 large tomato, roughly chopped into big chunks
16 black olives
splash of sherry vinegar
small handful of mint leaves, to serve – optional

This is a great summer dish and is brilliant on a barbecue. The fresh crispness of the salad cuts through the richness of the meat. If you want to change it up, beef mince works well with this recipe too.

METHOD

Preheat your grill to maximum.

Tip the lamb mince into a bowl. Add the cinnamon and cumin, spring onions, garlic and a generous pinch of salt and pepper, then mix the whole lot together thoroughly – I find the best way is to dig your hands in there.

Mould the mince mixture into 4 equal-sized sausage shapes around a skewer and place on your grill pan or a baking tray. Grill the koftas for 5 minutes on each side or until well browned and cooked through.

Meanwhile, toss the cucumber, tomato, olives and vinegar together in a bowl.

Serve your koftas with this chunky salad – and an artistic scattering of mint leaves, if you like.

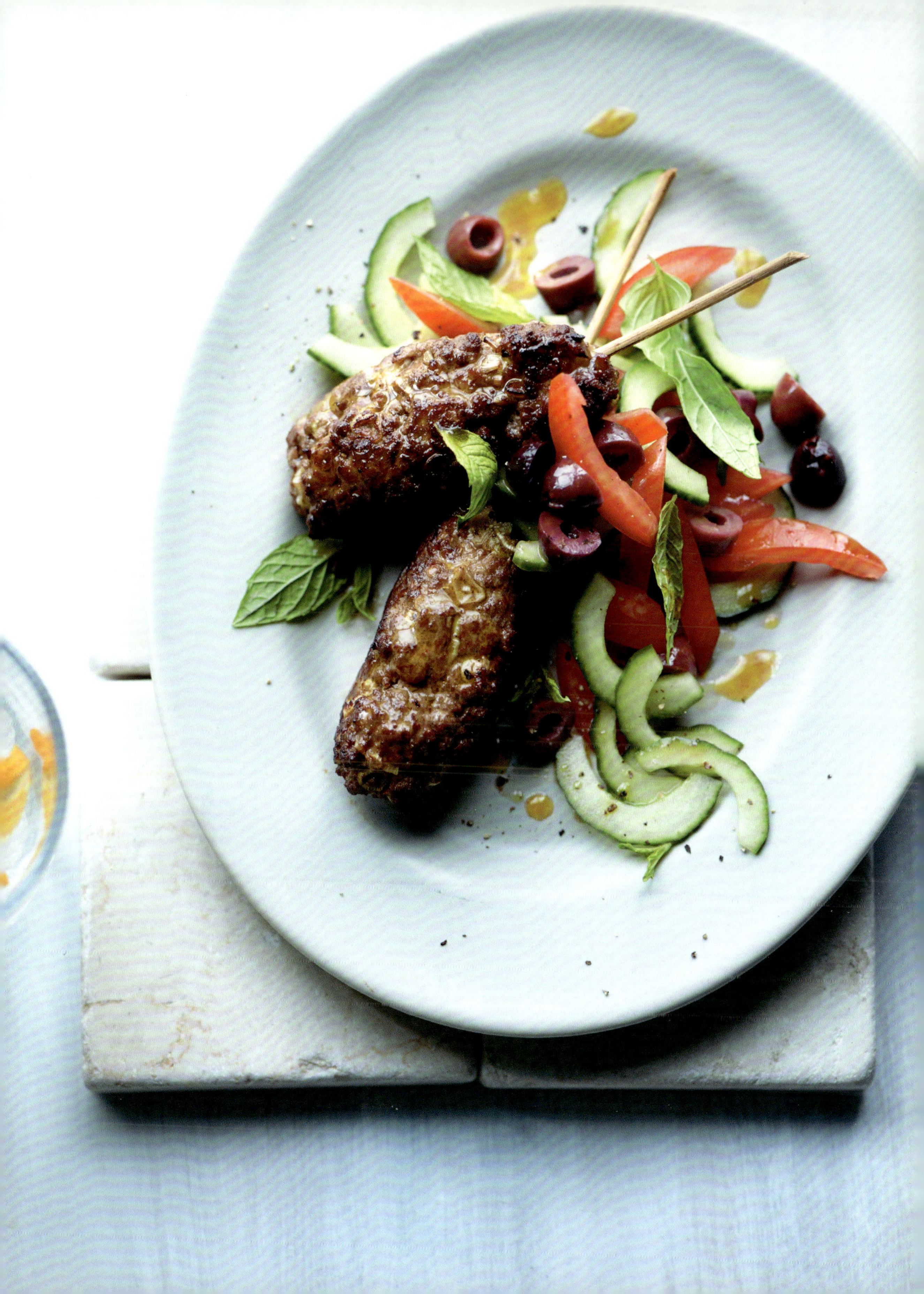

SERVES 4

COCONUT AND CASHEW DAAL

A lovely vegetarian option to try. This is going to take rather longer than most of my recipes (about an hour for this one), but it's time well spent, as it tastes amazing.

LONGER RECIPE
MAKE AHEAD
GOOD TO FREEZE

INGREDIENTS

- 250g yellow split peas (available in most supermarkets)
- 1 tbsp coconut oil
- 1 small red onion, roughly diced
- 1 tsp cumin seeds
- 1 cinnamon stick, broken in two
- 1 fresh bay leaf, or 2 dried
- 4 cloves garlic, finely chopped
- 5cm ginger, finely chopped
- 1 green chilli, split lengthways
- 1 tbsp garam masala
- 1 tsp ground turmeric
- 1 x 400ml tin of full-fat coconut milk
- 500ml warm vegetable stock
- 200g cashew nuts
- 2 large handfuls of baby spinach leaves
- bunch of coriander, leaves only, roughly chopped

METHOD

Place the split peas in a large bowl and cover with warm water from the tap. Leave to soak while you cook the onion and spices.

Melt the coconut oil in a large saucepan over a medium heat. Add the onion and cook for 3–4 minutes until just soft. Add the cumin seeds, cinnamon and bay leaves and stir-fry for 45 seconds, then add the garlic, ginger and chilli and cook for 1 minute. Sprinkle in the garam masala and turmeric powder and stir-fry for 30 seconds.

Drain the split peas and add to the pan, along with the coconut milk and half of the vegetable stock. Bring to the boil and simmer for about 30 minutes or until the split peas are completely tender.

Meanwhile, pour the rest of the vegetable stock over the cashew nuts and leave to soak for 10 minutes. Tip the nuts and stock into a blender and blitz until smooth.

When the split peas are tender, add the cashew cream and the spinach, then stir until the spinach has wilted into the daal. Remove from the heat and stir through the coriander before gobbling down your yummy daal.

★ Serve with a big portion of your favourite greens such as spinach, kale, broccoli, mange tout or green beans.

TURKEY MOUSSAKA

SERVES 4

LONGER RECIPE
MAKE AHEAD
GOOD TO FREEZE

INGREDIENTS

- 3 aubergines, cut lengthways into slices about 5mm thick
- about 100ml olive oil
- salt and pepper
- 1 large red onion, diced
- 3 cloves garlic, finely chopped
- 1kg turkey mince
- 1 tsp ground cinnamon
- 1 tbsp tomato puree
- 300ml chicken stock
- 2 tsp dried oregano
- 2 balls of mozzarella (about 250g)
- 4 tbsp finely grated parmesan
- bunch of parsley, leaves only, roughly chopped

Grilled aubergine is hard to beat – and in this moussaka, it becomes perfect dinner-party fodder. Even better, it can all be done in advance, so it's fuss-free. This dish actually takes more like 1 hour and 15 minutes to make, but for much of that time it looks after itself in the oven.

METHOD

Preheat your grill to maximum. Lay a single layer of aubergine slices on your grill pan or a baking tray, drizzle with a little olive oil and season with salt and pepper. Slide under the grill and cook for 2 minutes on each side. When cooked (soft to the touch and looking a little shrivelled), transfer the aubergine slices to a plate and repeat the process until they are all cooked and sitting happily on the plate.

Heat a splash of olive oil in a large saucepan over a medium to high heat. Add the onion and garlic and stir-fry for 3–4 minutes until beginning to soften. Increase the heat to high and add the turkey mince, cinnamon, tomato puree, chicken stock and oregano. Bring the whole lot up to the boil and leave to simmer for 20 minutes.

Preheat your oven to 190°C (fan 170°C, gas mark 5).

Pour about a quarter of the mince mixture into a deep baking dish. Tear up half a ball of mozzarella and scatter over the mince, then lay a third of the grilled aubergine slices on top (it doesn't matter if they overlap slightly). Repeat the process until you have 3 layers of mince and 3 layers of aubergine, then finish with the final quarter of the mince.

Scatter the parmesan over the top and cook the moussaka in the oven for about 30 minutes until heated through and golden brown. To finish your dish, sprinkle over the fresh parsley.

JOE'S CHICKEN PIE

SERVES 4

LONGER RECIPE
MAKE AHEAD
GOOD TO FREEZE

INGREDIENTS

- 2 large knobs of butter
- 1 large leek, washed and chopped into 2cm pieces
- 200g mushrooms, roughly chopped
- 4 x 250g chicken breast fillets, cut into bite-sized pieces
- 250ml chicken stock
- 1 tbsp cornflour
- 100ml double cream
- 2 large handfuls of baby spinach leaves
- about 6 sheets of filo pastry
- drizzle of olive oil
- salad or veg, to serve

If you love chicken pie, this recipe won't disappoint. It's actually Lean in about 60 minutes, but is such a nice treat that you won't mind the extra effort. Plus, there's cream and butter in it, so you know it's going to taste incredible.

METHOD

Preheat your oven to 190°C (fan 170°C, gas mark 5).

Heat the butter in a large frying pan over a medium to high heat. Add the leek and mushrooms and fry for 2–3 minutes until they just start to soften. Crank up the heat to high, add the chicken pieces and fry for a further 2 minutes – the chicken won't be cooked through at this point – then pour in the chicken stock and let it come to a simmer.

Meanwhile, mix the cornflour with 2 tablespoons of water until smooth, then pour into the pan, along with the cream. Bring back to the boil, stirring gently, and cook until the sauce thickens. Remove from the heat and stir in the spinach, then tip the whole lot into a pie dish about 28cm x 15cm. Set aside to cool a little.

Take a sheet of filo and roughly crumple it in your hands – there is no right or wrong to this method! Place the crumpled filo on top of the chicken filling in the pie dish and repeat with the remaining filo sheets.

Drizzle the pastry with olive oil, then bake the pie for about 20 minutes, by which time the filo will have crisped up and turned golden brown in places.

Serve up your pie with fresh salad or some vegetables.

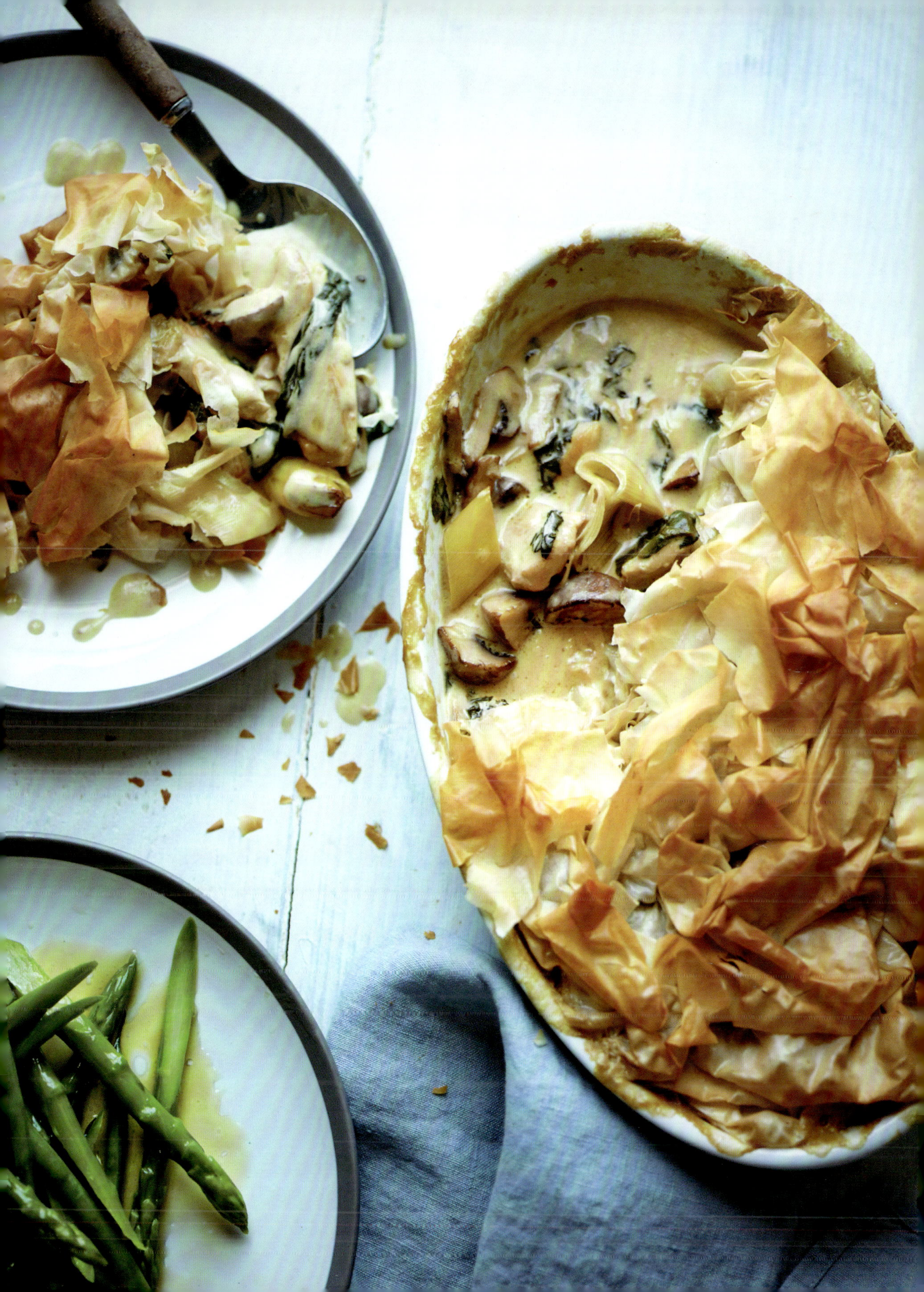

4

POST-WORKOUT CARBOHYDRATE-REFUEL RECIPES

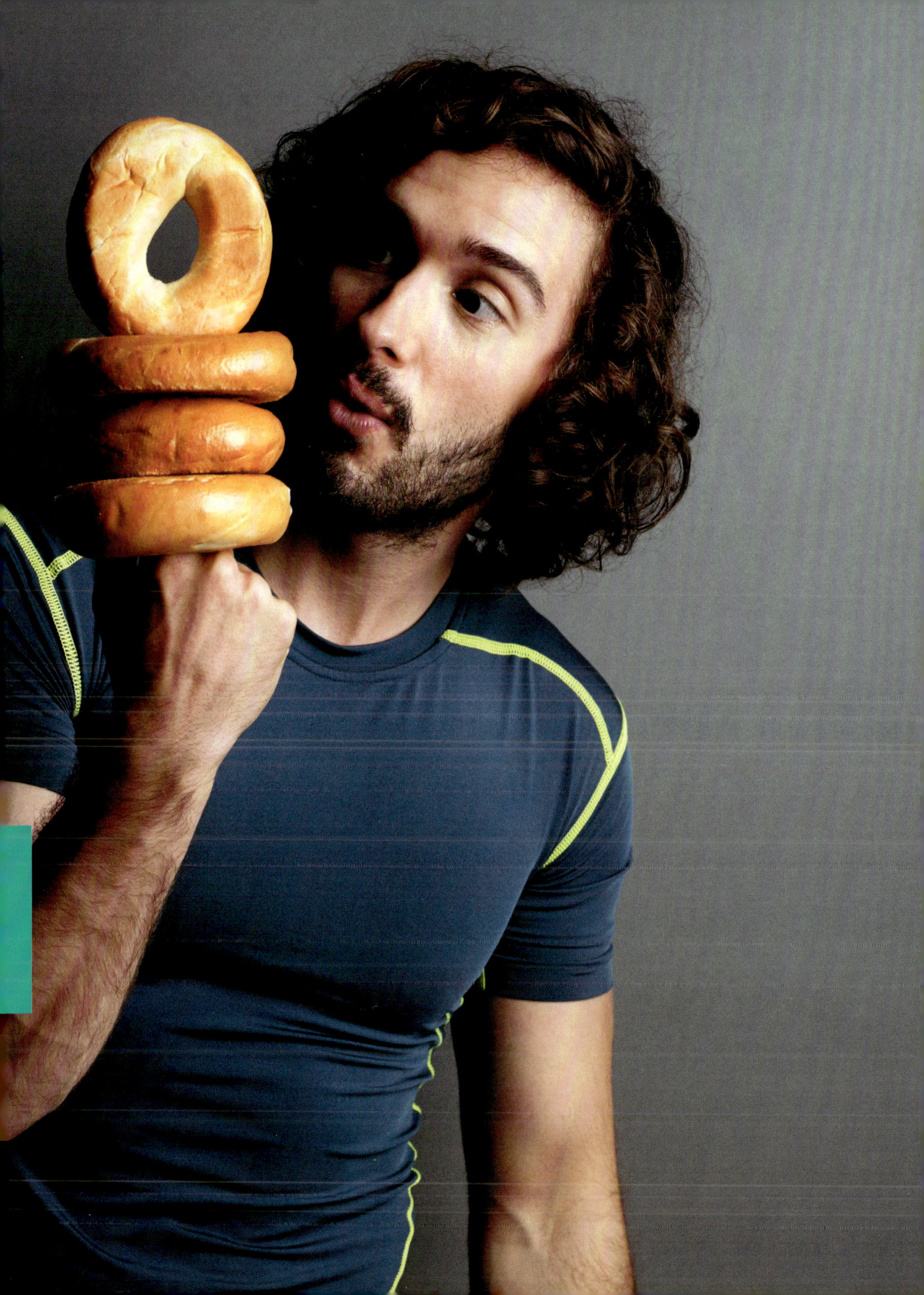

BANANA AND BLUEBERRY OVERNIGHT OATS

SERVES 1

This is a quick and easy breakfast to have ready to go, after jump-starting your day with a morning workout.

INGREDIENTS

- 1 banana, roughly chopped
- 75g full-fat yoghurt
- 250ml almond milk
- 1 scoop (30g) strawberry protein powder
- 100g rolled oats
- handful of pistachios or other nuts, blueberries and raspberries to serve

METHOD

Place the banana, yoghurt, almond milk and protein powder into a blender and blend until smooth. Pour the mixture into a bowl and stir in the oats, then cover and refrigerate for at least 4 hours, preferably overnight.

When ready to eat, top with the nuts, blueberries and raspberries.

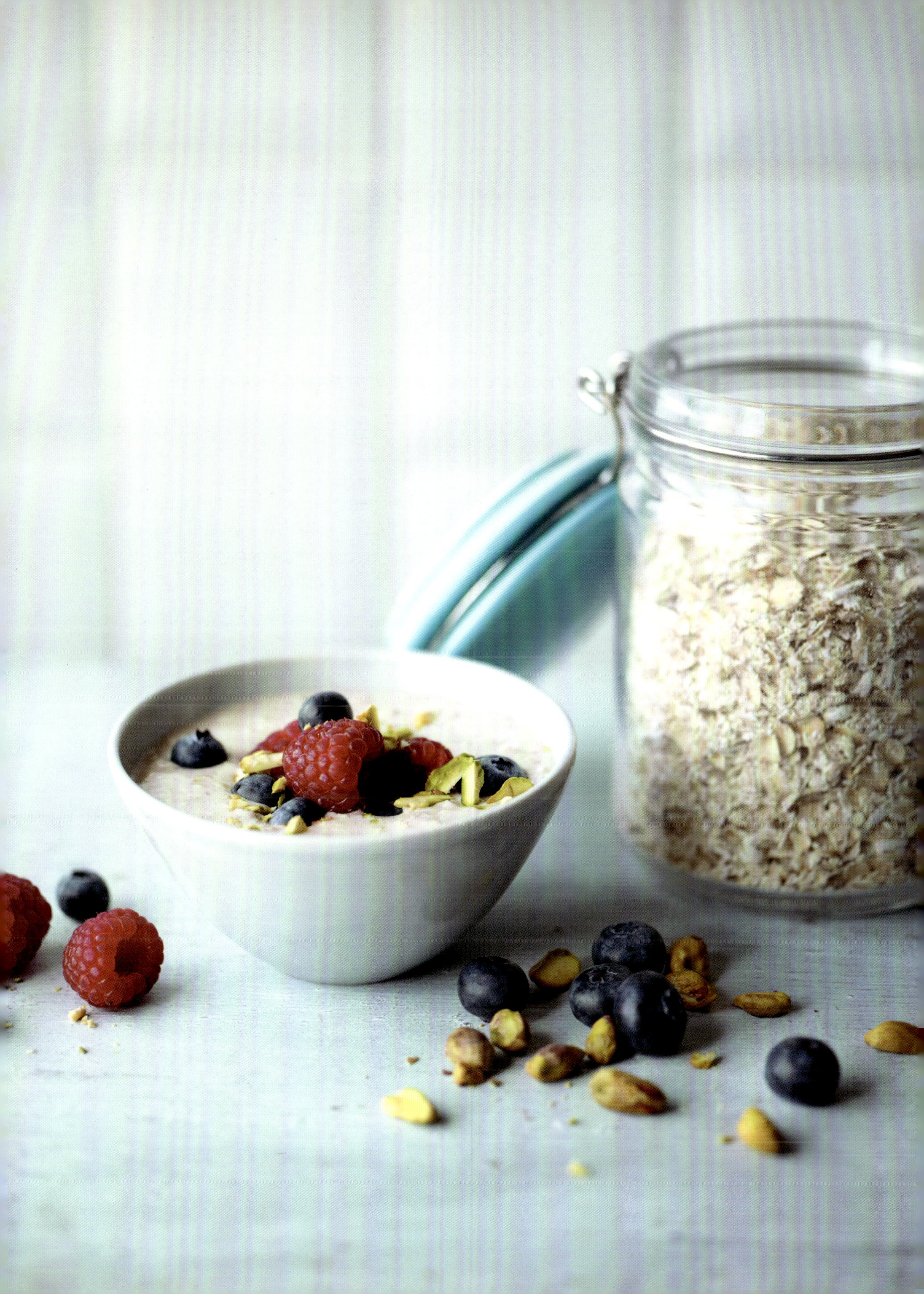

BIG McLEAN MUFFIN

SERVES 1

The thought of one of these waiting for you once you've finished your workout is enough to get you through those last reps. For the best poached eggs, use the freshest eggs possible.

INGREDIENTS

- 2 eggs
- 2 tsp coconut oil
- 5 cherry tomatoes
- 2 massive handfuls of baby spinach leaves
- 1 large English muffin
- 240g deli-style sliced ham or gammon, trimmed of visible fat
- 1 red chilli, finely sliced – optional

METHOD

Bring a saucepan of water to the boil. Carefully crack your eggs into the hot water, reducing the heat until the water is just 'burping'. Cook the eggs for about 4 minutes for runny yolks, then carefully lift them out with a slotted spoon and drain on paper towels.

Meanwhile, heat the coconut oil in a large frying pan over a medium to high heat. Add the tomatoes and toss in the hot oil for 1–2 minutes or until they are lightly browned and blistered. At this point, throw in the spinach and toss with the tomatoes until wilted, then remove the pan from the heat.

Toast your muffin, top with the ham or gammon and spoon over the tomatoes and spinach, then finish with the poached eggs and some sliced red chilli, if using.

WINNER'S PROTEIN PANCAKES

SERVES 1

Oooh, I can eat pancakes and get lean? Yes please – sold! These may look naughty, but they're actually the perfect post-workout treat, so stack 'em up and enjoy. You've earned them!

INGREDIENTS

1 banana, roughly chopped
1 scoop (30g) vanilla protein powder
1 egg
25g rolled oats
1 tbsp coconut oil
full-fat Greek yoghurt, blueberries and raspberries, to serve

METHOD

Whizz up the banana, protein powder, egg and oats in a blender to make your batter.

Heat up half the coconut oil in a non-stick frying pan over a medium heat. Pour little puddles of batter into the pan – I usually get 3 pancakes, with about half the batter in the pan at once. Cook for about 1 minute on each side. Remove and repeat the process with the rest of the batter.

Serve with a dollop of yoghurt and a few berries (see picture overleaf).

SERVES
1

BLUEBERRY AND BANANA PROTEIN SHAKE

INGREDIENTS

- 75g rolled oats
- large handful of blueberries
- handful of ice cubes
- 1 banana, roughly chopped
- 1 scoop (30g) vanilla or strawberry protein powder
- 1 tbsp chia seeds
- 250ml coconut water or water

This is a great way to get a load of vitamins into your diet, as it's so easy to make and transport (you can have it on your morning commute). I really recommend a good blender: they're worth their weight in gold. Just remember that protein shakes are fine to have now and then, but they aren't meant to replace actual food – so keep mixing it up!

METHOD

Place all the ingredients in a blender and blend until smooth.

★ TOP TIP

Chia seeds were an important food for the Aztecs and Mayans back in the day. They prized them for their ability to provide sustainable energy – in fact, 'chia' is the ancient Mayan word for 'strength'. Don't be fooled by their size! As a good source of fibre, protein and antioxidants, these little seeds pack a nutritional power punch.

SERVES
1

INCREDIBLE HULK SMOOTHIE

INGREDIENTS

- 200ml almond milk
- 1 granny smith apple, cored and roughly chopped
- 2 large handfuls (120g) of baby spinach leaves
- 1 scoop (30g) vanilla protein powder
- 75g rolled oats

This is green and good for you. I like to leave the skin on my apple, as it is full of nutrients, but you may prefer not to – either way is fine! Enjoy.

METHOD

Place all the ingredients in a blender with a handful of ice and blitz until smooth.

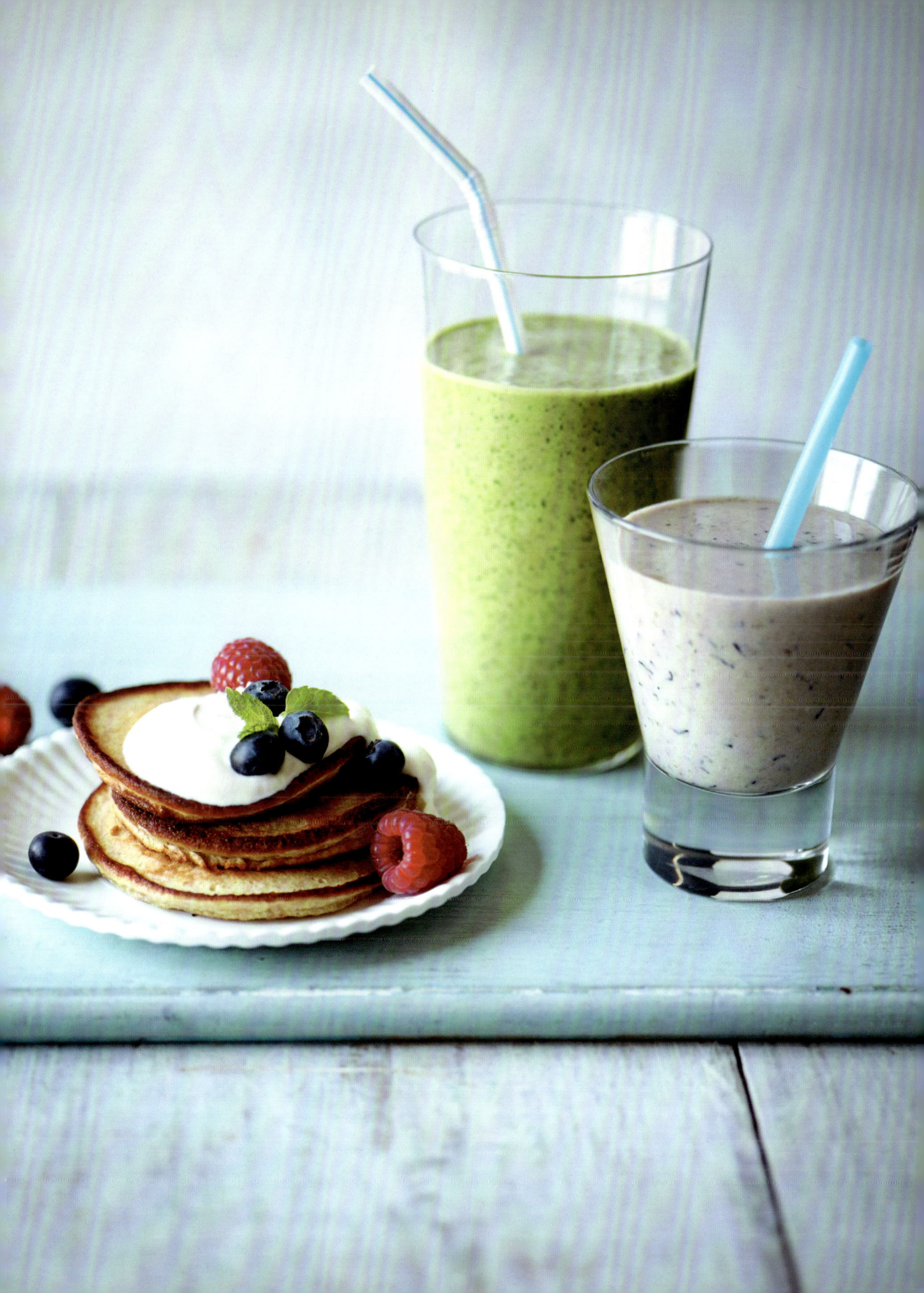

BUILD-UP BAGEL

Long live the build-up bagel. For some reason, people on my plan go absolutely bonkers for this post-workout bagel. I think they feel naughty eating it – but, like I say, you've just trained and earned those carbs, so no need to feel guilty. Go for good-quality cooked meat, not the nasty cheap re-formed stuff. If you don't want to bother with poaching the egg, you could always just boil and slice it instead.

SERVES 1

INGREDIENTS

1 egg
1 plain bagel
2 tsp chipotle paste or barbecue sauce
1 tbsp full-fat Greek yoghurt
large handful of rocket
1 tomato, sliced
150g deli-style cooked turkey or chicken breast
75g deli-style sliced roast beef

METHOD

Bring a saucepan of water to the boil. Carefully crack your egg into the hot water, reducing the heat until the water is just 'burping'. Cook the egg for about 4 minutes for a runny yolk, then carefully lift it out with a slotted spoon and drain on paper towels.

Slice the bagel in half and toast it for a couple of minutes.

Spread the toasted bagel evenly with the chipotle paste or barbecue sauce and the yoghurt, and then begin building your bagel: start with the rocket and tomato, followed by the turkey or chicken and the beef, then the poached egg. Finally, stick the top on the bagel and get munching!

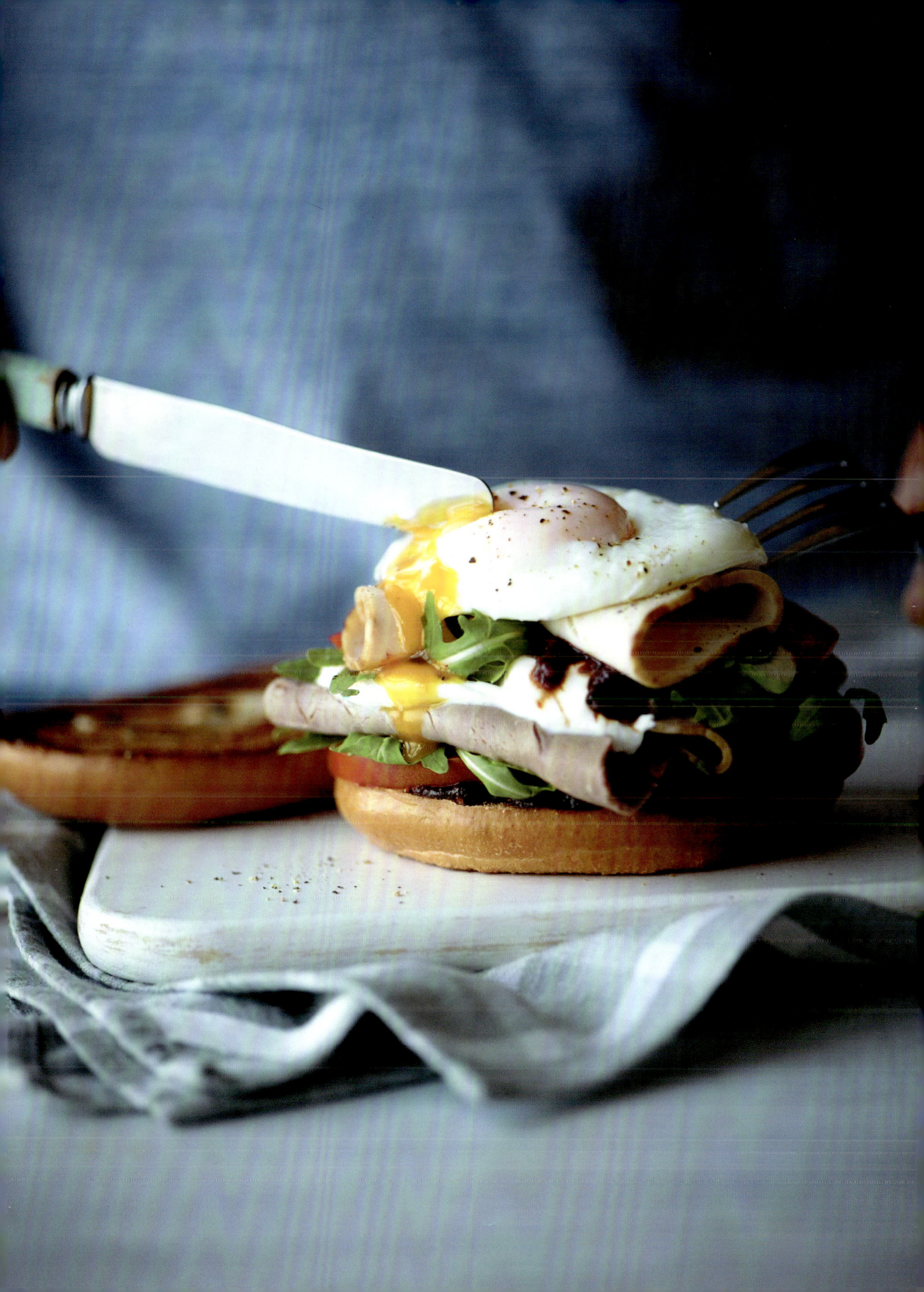

CHICKEN AND NEW POTATO HASH

SERVES 1

Standing around waiting for potatoes to boil? No, thanks. Bang them in the microwave instead and cook them in half the time. This is proper comfort food – a real reward after a workout. You won't feel hungry after this one.

INGREDIENTS

200g new potatoes
½ tbsp coconut oil
1 x 200g skinless chicken breast fillet, sliced into 1cm thick strips
4 spring onions, sliced
75g mange tout
1 egg
1 tsp smoked paprika
2 large handfuls of baby spinach leaves
pinch of chilli flakes, if you like it hot

METHOD

Prick the new potatoes with a fork and blast them in the microwave at 900w for 8 minutes.

Meanwhile, melt the oil in a large frying pan over a medium to high heat. Add the chicken and fry for 2 minutes, stirring occasionally – you want the chicken to be browned in places. Add the spring onions and the mange tout and stir-fry for 1 minute, then remove from the heat. You should now have about 4 minutes until your spuds ping, so time for a quick set of press-ups – go!

Bring a saucepan of water to the boil. Carefully crack your egg into the hot water, reducing the heat until the water is just 'burping'. Cook the egg for about 4 minutes for a runny yolk, then carefully lift it out with a slotted spoon and drain on paper towels.

Once the spuds have pinged, carefully (maybe using a knife and fork, as they'll be very hot) halve them, cutting any larger ones into quarters. Return the frying pan to a high heat, then slide in the potatoes and fry, without turning, for about 3–4 minutes or until the potatoes are beginning to brown in places. Add the smoked paprika and spinach, then toss to coat all the ingredients evenly and wilt the spinach.

Spoon up your hash, top with the poached egg and finish with a little chilli flake fire, if you want.

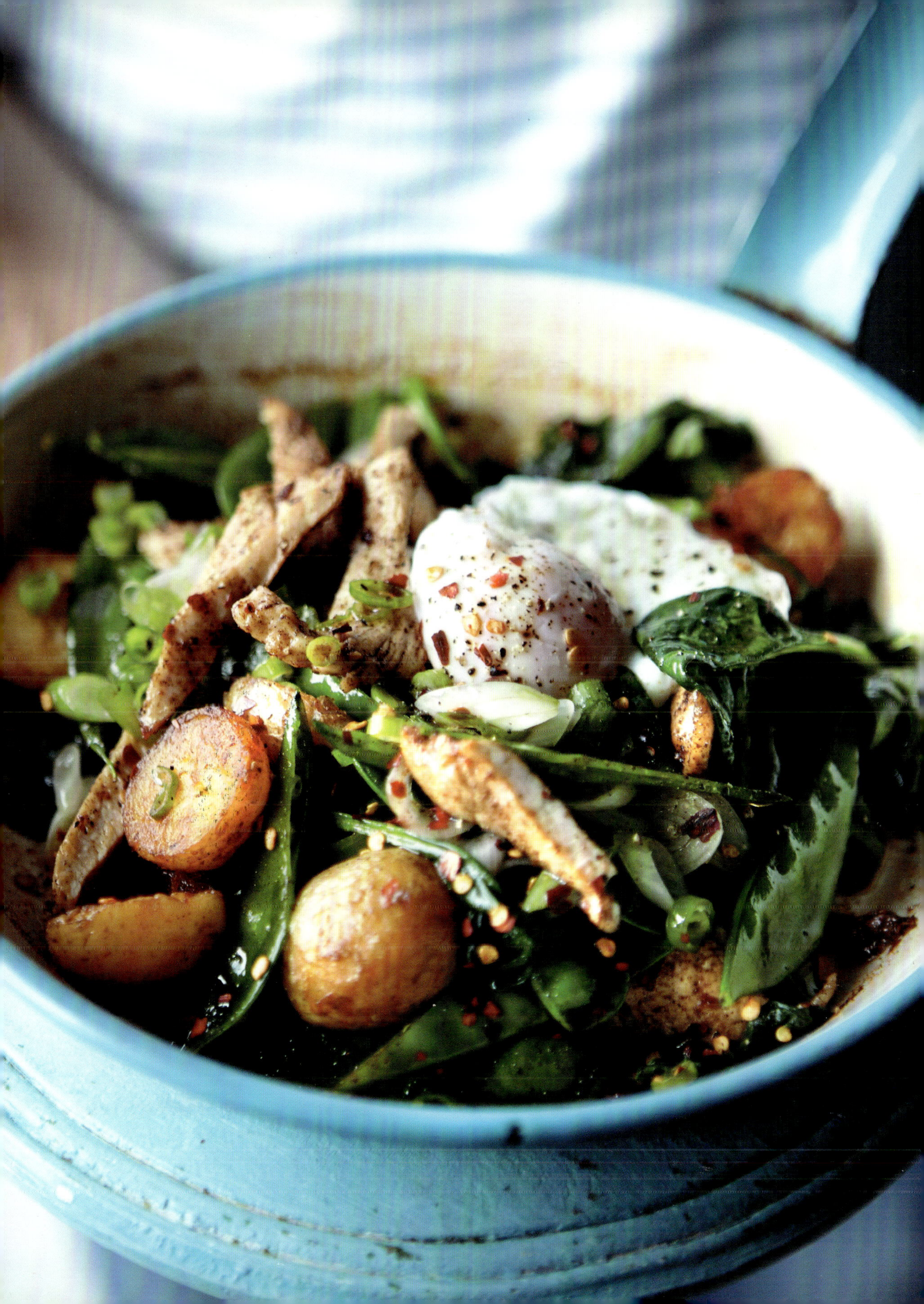

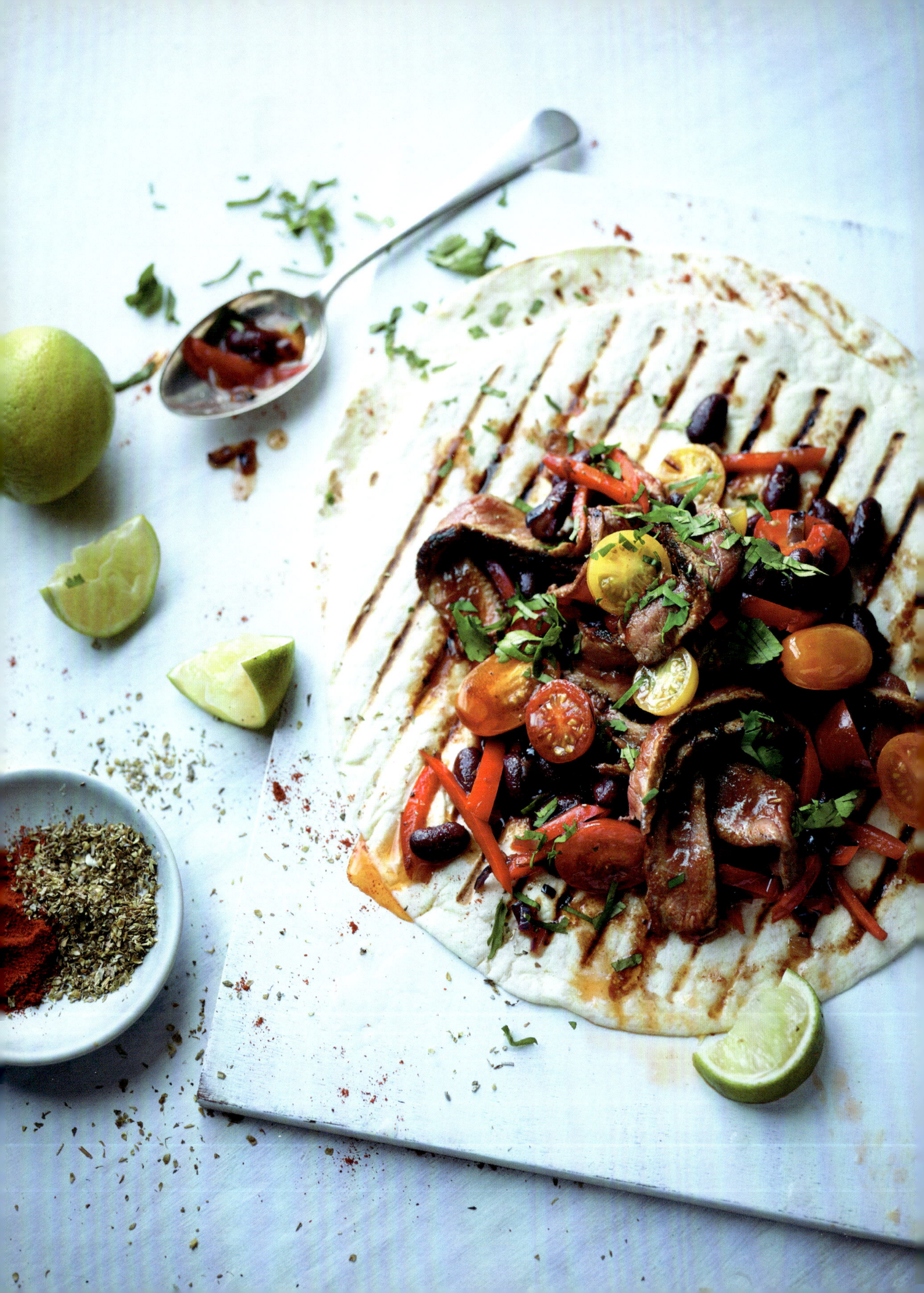

BAD-BOY BURRITO

SERVES 2

You've just worked out and earned your carbs. This monster burrito needs two hands to eat, and is a proper treat that's guaranteed to fill you up and leave you feeling like a hero. It's also really quick and easy to make up and then carry with you to work. For a change, try using chicken instead of beef, or pitta bread instead of tortillas.

MAKE AHEAD

INGREDIENTS

1 tbsp coconut oil
500g sirloin steak, trimmed of visible fat and cut into 1cm thick slices
1 red onion, roughly chopped
1 red pepper, de-seeded and roughly sliced
1 clove garlic, finely chopped
1 tsp paprika
1 tsp dried oregano
6 cherry tomatoes, roughly chopped
salt and pepper
1 x 400g tin of kidney beans, drained and rinsed
2 large tortilla wraps
small bunch of coriander, leaves only, roughly chopped
squeeze of lime juice

METHOD

Heat the coconut oil in a large frying pan over a high heat. Add the steak and fry for 1–2 minutes, turning the meat a couple of times. Throw in the onion, red pepper and garlic and stir-fry for a minute or two. Add the paprika, oregano and tomatoes, season with salt and pepper, and toss everything together for a minute. Chuck in the kidney beans and cook for another minute, by which time the beans should be warmed through.

Pile half the mixture along the middle of each wrap, then top with some chopped coriander and finish with a squeeze of lime juice. Roll up and gobble down.

SERVES 1

MAKE AHEAD
(the chilli not the sweet potato)

INGREDIENTS

1 sweet potato
2 tsp coconut oil
3 spring onions, finely sliced
250g reduced-fat (about 5%) beef mince
1 tsp ground cumin
1 tsp smoked paprika
2 tsp tomato puree
175g tinned kidney beans, drained and rinsed
100ml beef stock
1 tbsp full-fat Greek yoghurt

SWEET POTATO WITH CHILLI

Sweet potato is one of my favourite carb sources and when you combine it with a quick beef chilli, it's a real banger. To make this Lean in 15, I use a microwave to cook the potato, but if you'd rather boil the sweet potato or bake it in the oven, go for it.

METHOD

Prick the sweet potato a couple of times with a fork, then blast it in the microwave at 900w for 5 minutes. Leave it to rest for 30 seconds and then blast it for a further 3–4 minutes. Set aside, loosely covered in foil, until needed.

Meanwhile, melt the coconut oil in a large frying pan over a high heat. Stir in the spring onions and beef and stir-fry for about 4 minutes, breaking up any chunks of mince as you go. When the meat is browned, sprinkle in the cumin and paprika and cook for 30 seconds before squeezing in the tomato puree. Stir-fry for another 30 seconds, then add the kidney beans and beef stock. Bring to a simmer and cook for 1 minute.

Split open the sweet potato and serve with the quick chilli – and some cooling yoghurt.

★ Serve with a big portion of your favourite greens such as spinach, kale, broccoli, mange tout or green beans.

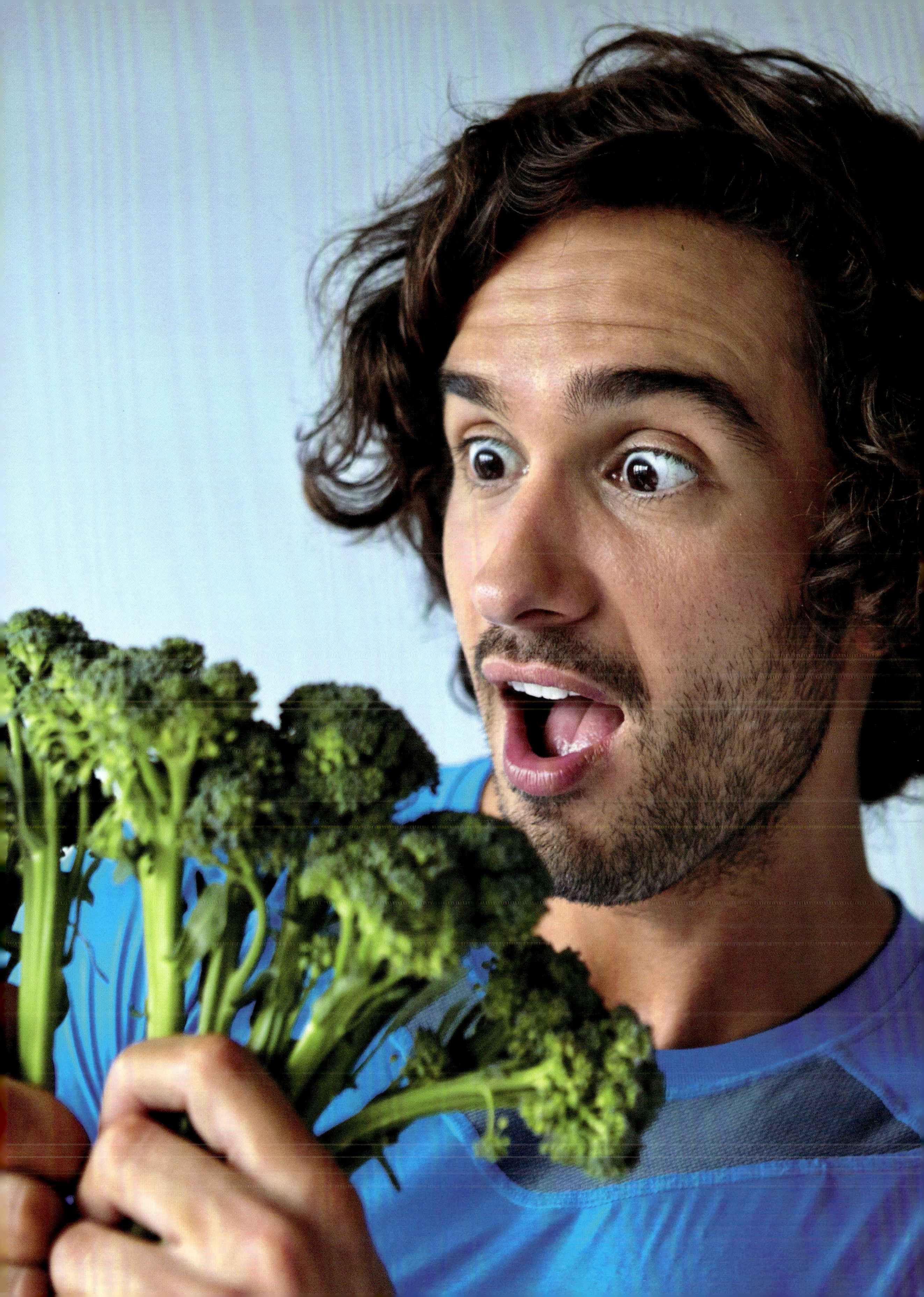

PRAWN AND NOODLE STIR-FRY

SERVES 1

MAKE AHEAD

INGREDIENTS

½ tbsp coconut oil
3 spring onions, finely sliced
1 clove garlic, finely chopped
200g raw prawns, peeled
50g mange tout, sliced in half
3 baby sweetcorn, sliced in half
4 midget trees (tender-stem broccoli), any bigger stalks sliced in half lengthways
200g 'straight to wok' noodles
2 tbsp light soy sauce
1 tbsp fish sauce

This is about as lean as they come. One wok, no hassle and another chance to throw some midget trees around. This makes a great lunch, too, so cook double and take the extra in a lunch box to work the next day.

METHOD

Melt the coconut oil in a wok or large frying pan over a medium to high heat. Add the spring onions and garlic and stir-fry for 1 minute. Add the prawns and continue to stir for a further minute.

Toss in the mange tout, sweetcorn and midget trees, along with about 2 tablespoons of water. Let the water bubble up and create steam to cook the vegetables. Add the noodles, breaking up the clumps with your fingers as you drop them in. Toss to mix the noodles with the other ingredients, then stir-fry for a minute until the noodles are warmed through and soft.

Remove from the heat, pour in the soy sauce and fish sauce, then give the whole lot one last stir before piling onto a plate and munching away.

★ TOP TIP

For a gluten-free meal, swap the soy sauce for tamari, and use rice noodles instead of the 'straight to wok' variety.

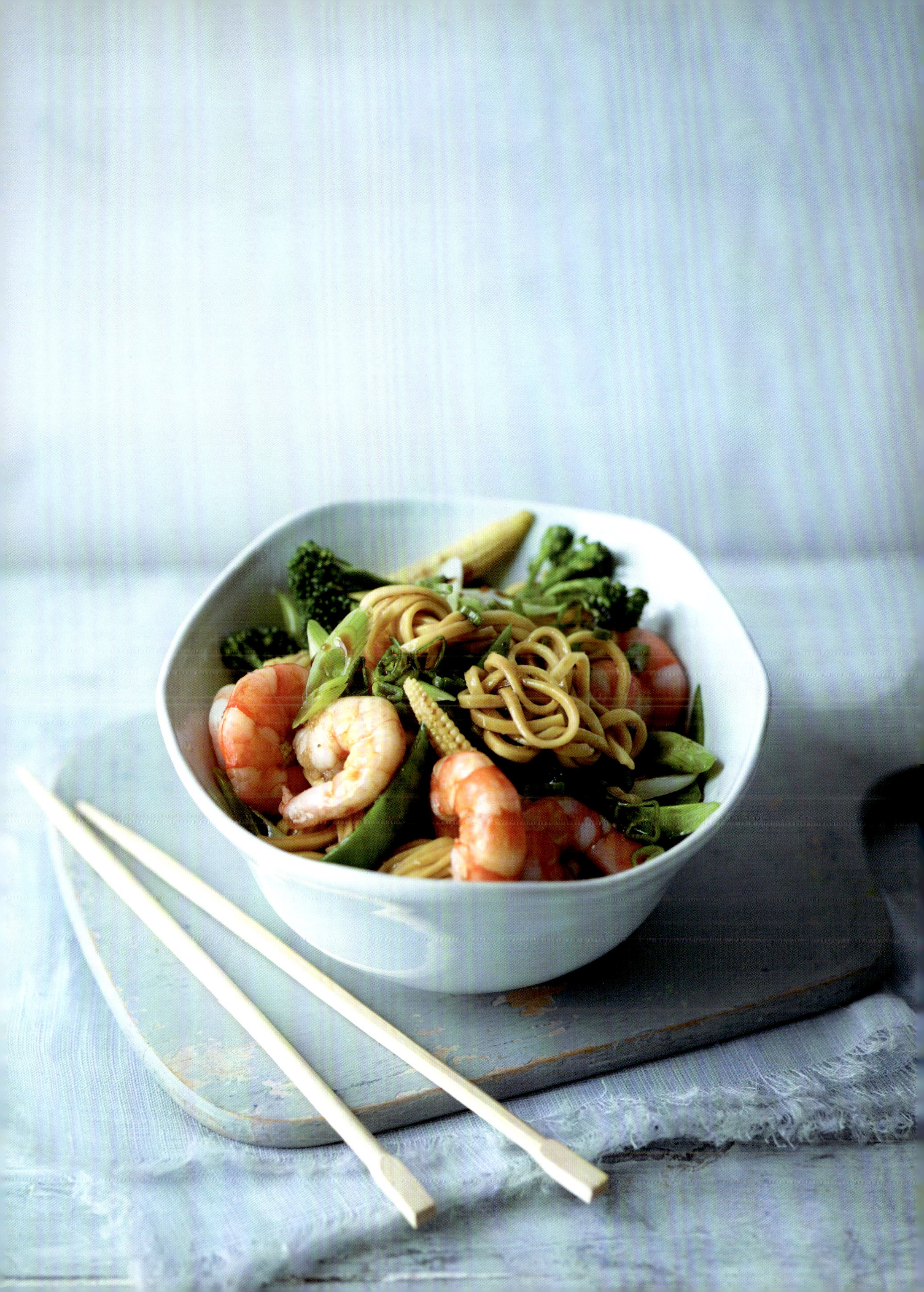

IN-A-HURRY CURRY FRIED RICE

SERVES 1

MAKE AHEAD

INGREDIENTS

1 tbsp coconut oil
1 small red onion, roughly diced
1 clove garlic, roughly diced
2cm ginger, roughly diced
250g skinless chicken breast fillet, sliced into 1cm thick strips
½ red pepper, de-seeded and sliced
1 tbsp mild curry powder
250g pre-cooked basmati rice
big handful of baby spinach leaves
squeeze of lime juice

If you're craving a curry and thinking of ordering a greasy takeaway, hold your horses and make this instead. It's lean, it tastes great and it will arrive quicker than any Indian takeaway. It tastes awesome with diced pork or turkey too.

METHOD

Melt the coconut oil in a wok or large frying pan over a medium to high heat. Add the onion and stir-fry for 1 minute, then add the garlic and ginger and cook for a further minute. Toss in the chicken, red pepper and half of the curry powder and stir-fry for 2 minutes.

Add the rice, crumbling it between your fingers as you drop it in, then pour in 2 tablespoons of water. Stir-fry for 2 minutes until the rice is warmed through and the chicken is completely cooked. Check by slicing into one of the larger pieces to make sure the meat is white all the way through, with no raw pink bits left.

Add the remaining curry powder, along with the spinach, and stir until the spinach has wilted slightly and the curry powder is evenly distributed.

Dish up your yummy curry fried rice, finishing with a big squeeze of lime juice.

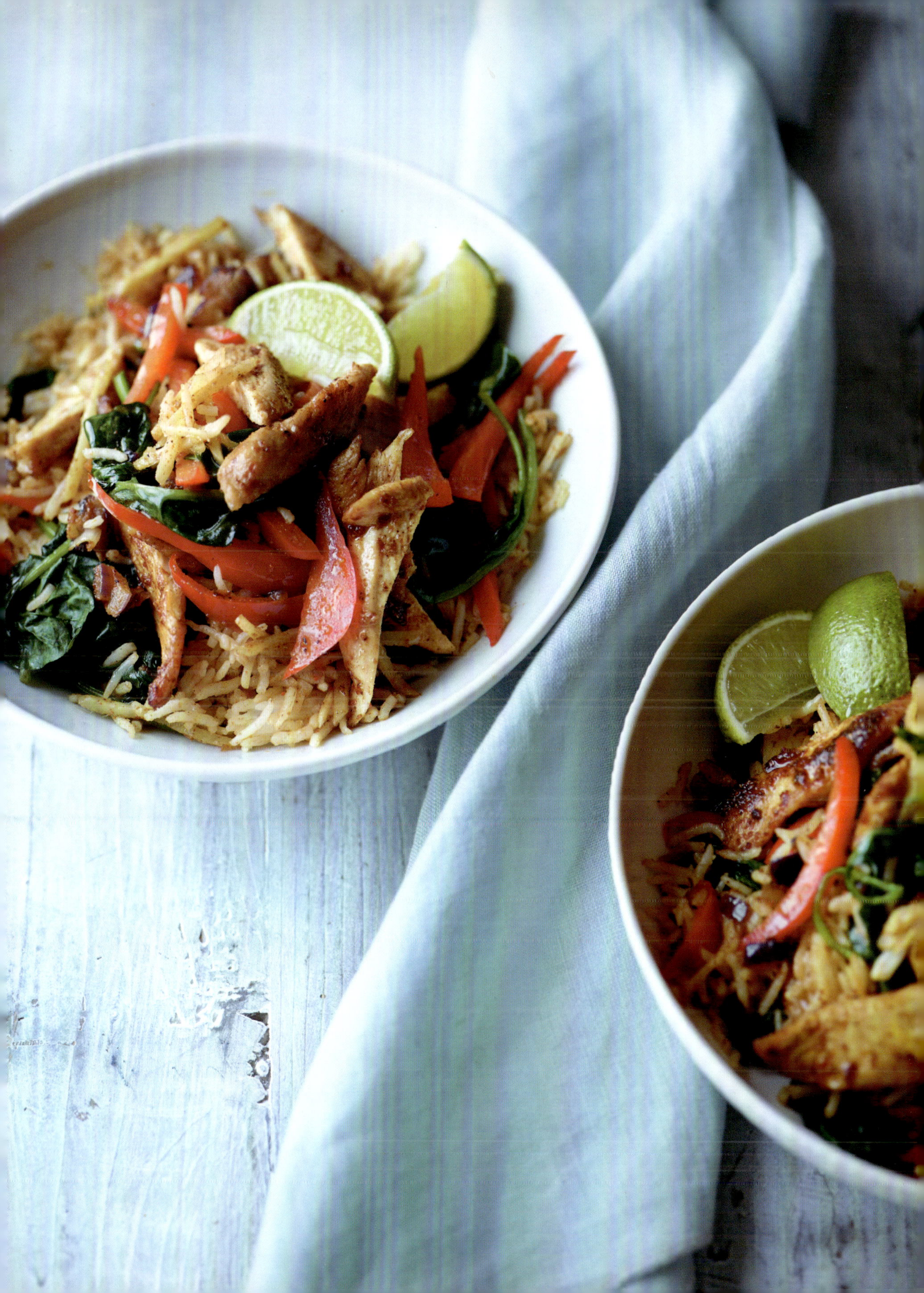

THE BODY COACH CLUB SANDWICH

SERVES 1

MAKE AHEAD

INGREDIENTS

- 2 eggs
- salt and pepper
- 4 slices of thick sliced bread
- 1 large tomato, sliced
- ½ round lettuce, leaves only
- 300g mixed sliced deli-style meats – I like turkey and ham
- 1 big pickled gherkin, to serve – optional

The Body Coach club sandwich is a beautiful thing! I've stuck with tradition and gone with turkey and ham, but feel free to improvise. And if the four-layer sandwich is too much for you, drop a layer and add a handful of sweet potato chips instead (see below).

METHOD

Bring a saucepan of water to the boil before carefully lowering in the eggs and boiling for 6 minutes. Drain, then run the eggs under cold water until cool enough to handle and peel them. Place the eggs in a small bowl, season generously with salt and pepper, then crush with the back of a fork.

Toast your bread. When the toast is ready, build up your sandwich: lay the 4 slices of toast in front of you, spread each one with the crushed egg, then divide the tomato, lettuce and meat evenly among 3 of the slices. Stack up these 3 slices, then flip the last one over to create a lid.

Slice into triangles and gobble down with a gherkin chaser.

★ TOP TIP

To make the sweet potato chips, slice a large sweet potato lengthways into 8 wedges. Microwave the wedges for 4 minutes at 900w, then leave to stand for 1 minute. Heat 1 tbsp of coconut oil and fry the par-cooked chips in the oil until brown and crisp all over. Drain on paper towels and season with salt.

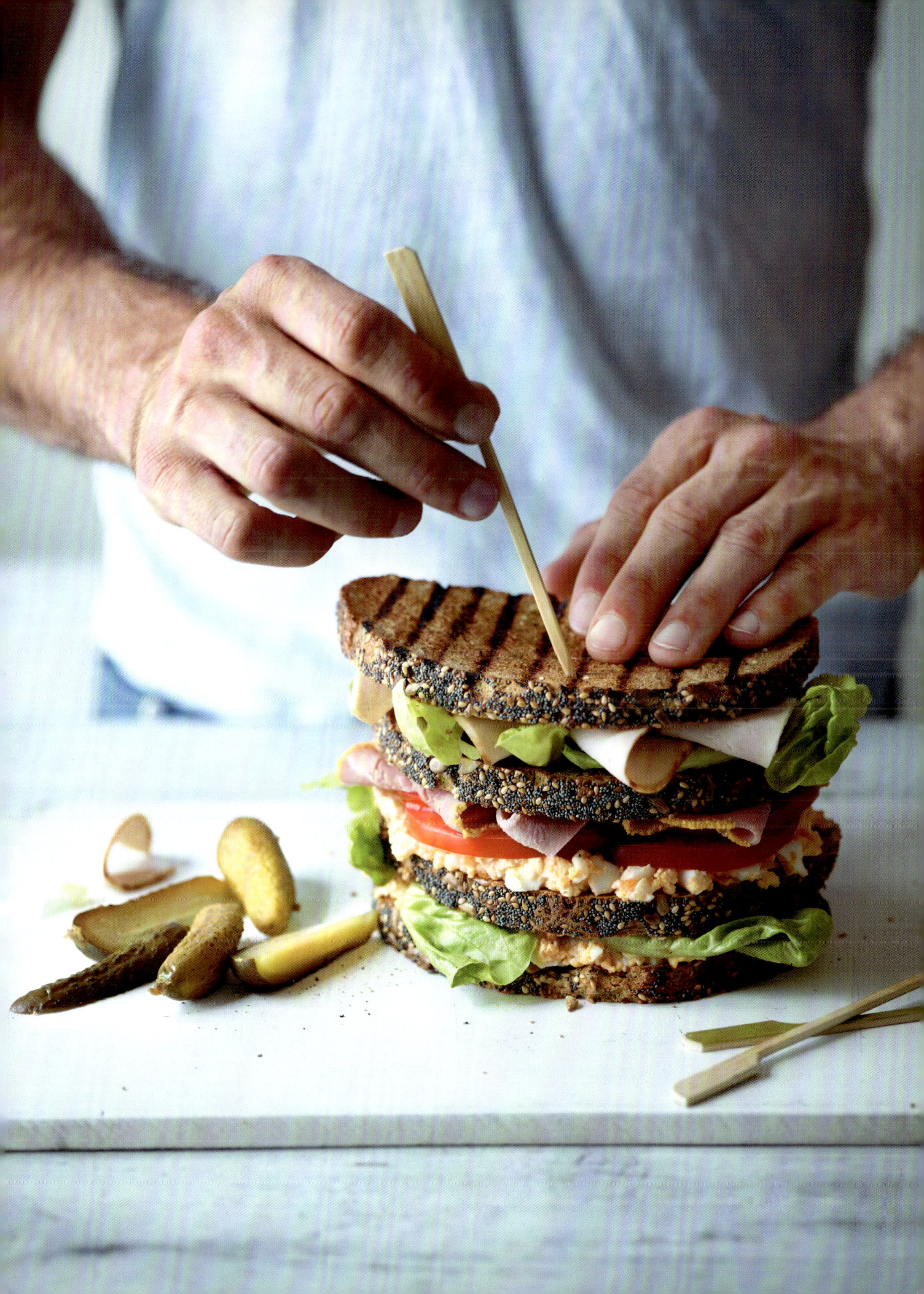

THAI BEEF STIR-FRY

SERVES 1

Fast and full of vibrant flavours, this will become a favourite. I predict you'll be eating this once a week when you've tried it. And if you become bored with egg noodles, try any of the 'straight to wok' types, or choose rice noodles for a gluten-free meal.

MAKE AHEAD

INGREDIENTS

½ tbsp coconut oil
2 star anise
1 bird's eye chilli, finely chopped – remove the seeds if you don't like it hot
2 cloves garlic, finely chopped
3 spring onions, finely sliced
1 lemongrass stalk, tender white part only, finely sliced
250g sirloin steak, trimmed of visible fat and sliced into 1cm thick strips
240g fresh egg noodles
2 tsp fish sauce
small bunch of coriander, leaves only, roughly chopped
juice of 1 lime

METHOD

Melt the coconut oil in a wok or large frying pan over a high heat. Add the star anise and leave to infuse the oil for 30 seconds, then remove. Add the chilli, garlic, spring onions and lemongrass and stir-fry for 1 minute.

Add the steak and stir-fry for a further 1–2 minutes until the beef is almost cooked.

Tumble in the noodles, along with a couple of tablespoons of water – this will create steam, helping to separate and warm the egg noodles. Toss everything together until you are satisfied that the beef is cooked and the noodles are warmed through.

Remove from the heat, add the fish sauce, coriander and lime juice, then serve up.

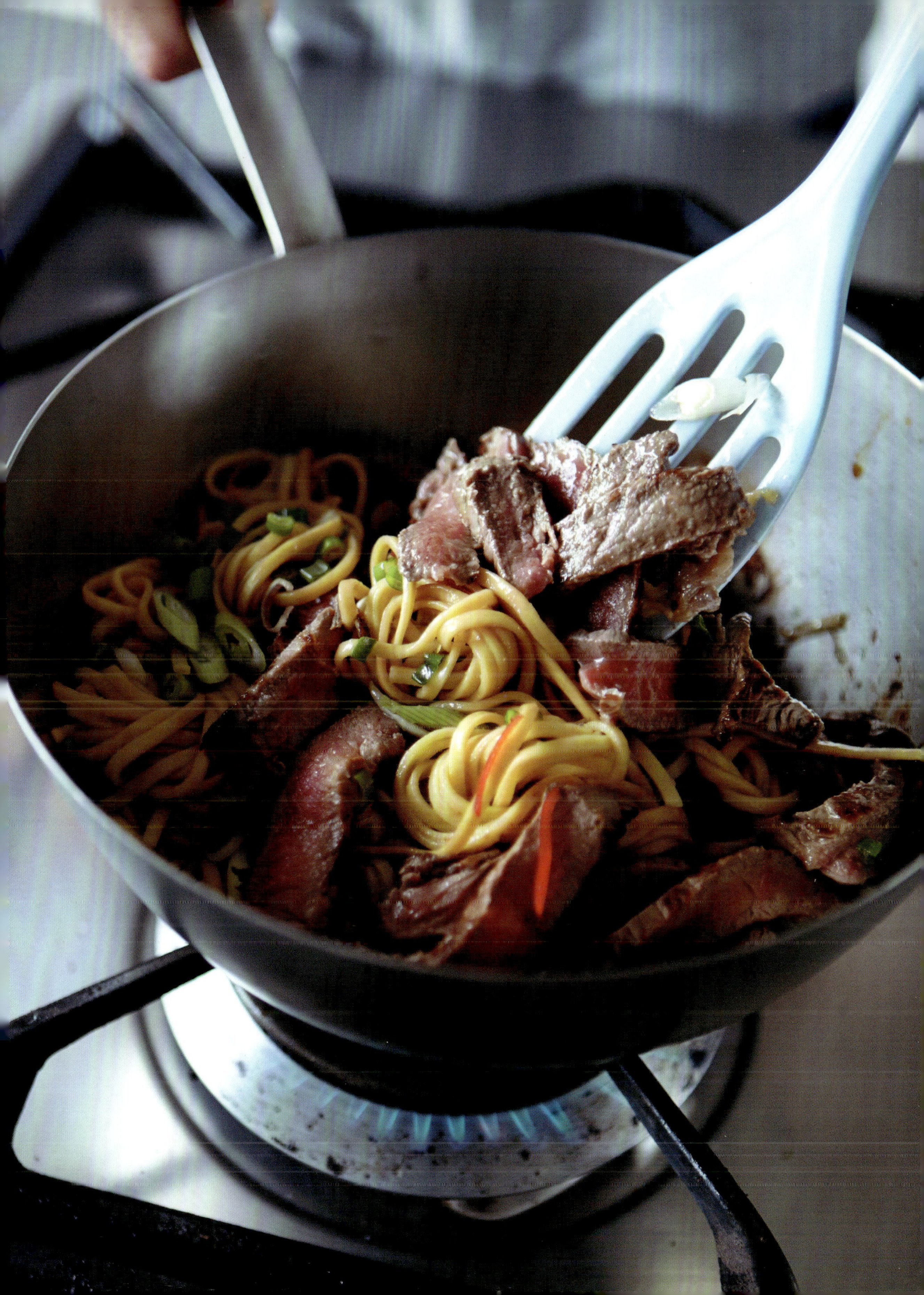

BAHN MI (VIETNAMESE PORK SANDWICH)

SERVES 1

MAKE AHEAD

INGREDIENTS

- ½ tbsp coconut oil
- ½ red onion, sliced into thin wedges
- 300g pork fillet, cut into 1cm thick slices
- 1 red chilli, sliced – remove the seeds if you don't like it hot
- 3 tsp fish sauce
- juice of 2 limes
- 2 tsp honey
- 2 tsp sesame oil
- ½ large baguette
- 1 tbsp chipotle paste
- 1 baby gem lettuce, leaves separated
- ¼ cucumber, sliced into thin batons
- mint and coriander leaves, to serve

This Vietnamese speciality uses pork loin, which is a great source of low-fat, inexpensive protein.

METHOD

Melt the coconut oil in a wok or frying pan over a medium to high heat. Add the onion and fry for 2 minutes or until starting to soften. Increase the heat to high, add the pork and chilli and stir-fry for 2–3 minutes, by which time the pork should be cooked through. Check by cutting into one of the larger pieces of meat to make sure there is no pink left. Remove the pan from the heat and pour in the fish sauce, lime juice, honey and sesame oil. Toss everything together until well mixed.

Cut the baguette in half lengthways and spread evenly with the chipotle paste. Build up your sandwich by laying lettuce leaves on the base, followed by the pork, cucumber and fresh herbs. Clamp the other half of the baguette on top and devour it.

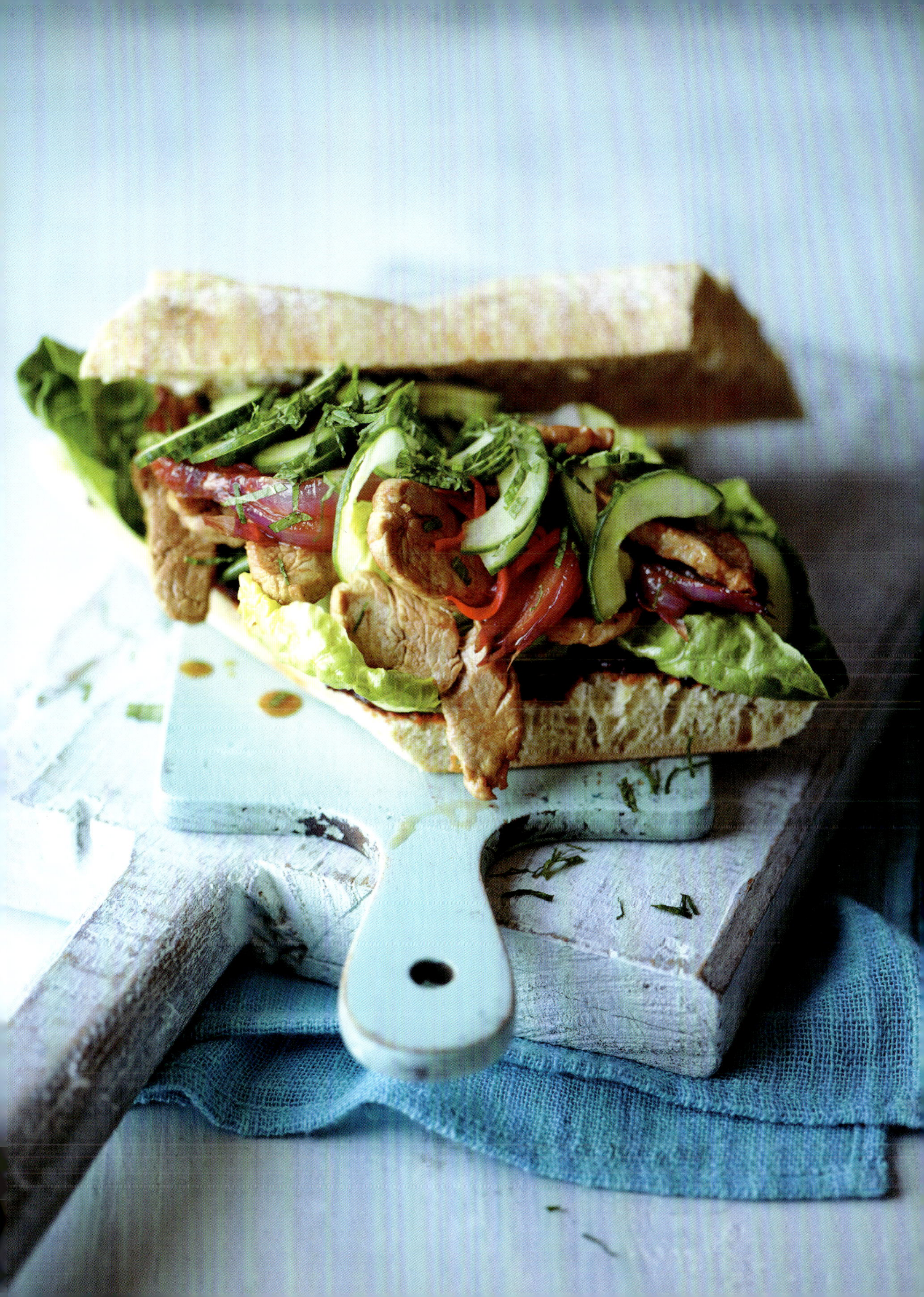

SAG ALOO WITH CHICKEN

SERVES 1

MAKE AHEAD

INGREDIENTS

250g new potatoes
½ tbsp coconut oil
4 spring onions, finely sliced
2 cloves garlic, finely chopped
2cm ginger, finely chopped
1 tbsp garam masala
1 x 240g skinless chicken breast fillet, sliced into 1cm thick strips
salt and pepper
2 large handfuls of baby spinach leaves
½ bunch of coriander, leaves only, roughly chopped
squeeze of lemon juice

Potatoes don't need to be bland and boring. This Indian-inspired dish tastes incredible and is much leaner than a greasy takeaway from your local curry house.

METHOD

Prick each potato once with a fork. Place in a microwave-proof bowl, pour over a splash of water and microwave for 2½ minutes at 900w, then leave to rest for 30 seconds before giving them a final 3-minute blast. Leave the potatoes to stand for a further 30 seconds, before carefully slicing them in half.

Melt the coconut oil in a wok or large frying pan over a medium to high heat. Add the spring onions, garlic and ginger and fry for 1 minute, stirring regularly. Tumble in the potatoes and mix in well. Sprinkle in the garam masala and fry for 30 seconds, stirring constantly – be careful not to let it catch. Quickly add the chicken, along with 2 tablespoons of water, to help cook the chicken and stop the spices burning. Season generously with salt and pepper and fry for 3–4 minutes, by which time the chicken should be cooked through. Check by slicing into one of the larger pieces to make sure the meat is white all the way through, with no raw pink bits left.

Add the spinach and toss through until wilted – there is no such thing as too much spinach at this point! Remove from the heat, sprinkle in the coriander and finish with a squeeze of lemon juice.

TURKEY AND CHICKPEA PITTAS

SERVES 1

MAKE AHEAD

INGREDIENTS

200g tinned chickpeas, drained and rinsed
½ tbsp coconut oil
½ red onion, diced
1 clove garlic, finely diced
250g turkey mince
2 tsp ground cumin
1 tsp smoked paprika
salt and pepper
1 carrot, grated
1 red chilli, finely sliced – remove the seeds if you don't like it hot
½ bunch of coriander, leaves only, roughly chopped
squeeze of lemon juice
2 pitta breads, to serve

The flavours in this dish remind me of falafel. If you don't have chickpeas, try making it with cannellini or butter beans. And, if you like, you can ditch the pitta and wrap it all up in a tortilla instead!

METHOD

Bring a saucepan of water to the boil, add the chickpeas and simmer for 5 minutes. Drain in a sieve or colander, then rinse under cold running water.

Meanwhile, heat the coconut oil in a large frying pan over a high heat. Add the onion and garlic and fry for 1 minute, then throw in the turkey mince and fry for 2 minutes, breaking up any big lumps as you go. Sprinkle in the cumin and paprika and fry for 30 seconds, by which time the turkey mince should be cooked. Season generously with salt and pepper, then stir in the carrot, chilli and chickpeas, using the back of your spoon to crush some of the chickpeas.

When you are happy that the turkey is fully cooked and the chickpeas are warmed through, remove the pan from the heat, stir through the chopped coriander and finish with a good squeeze of lemon juice. Load into pitta breads and eat.

Extra smoked pap
Add pepper as can be dry.

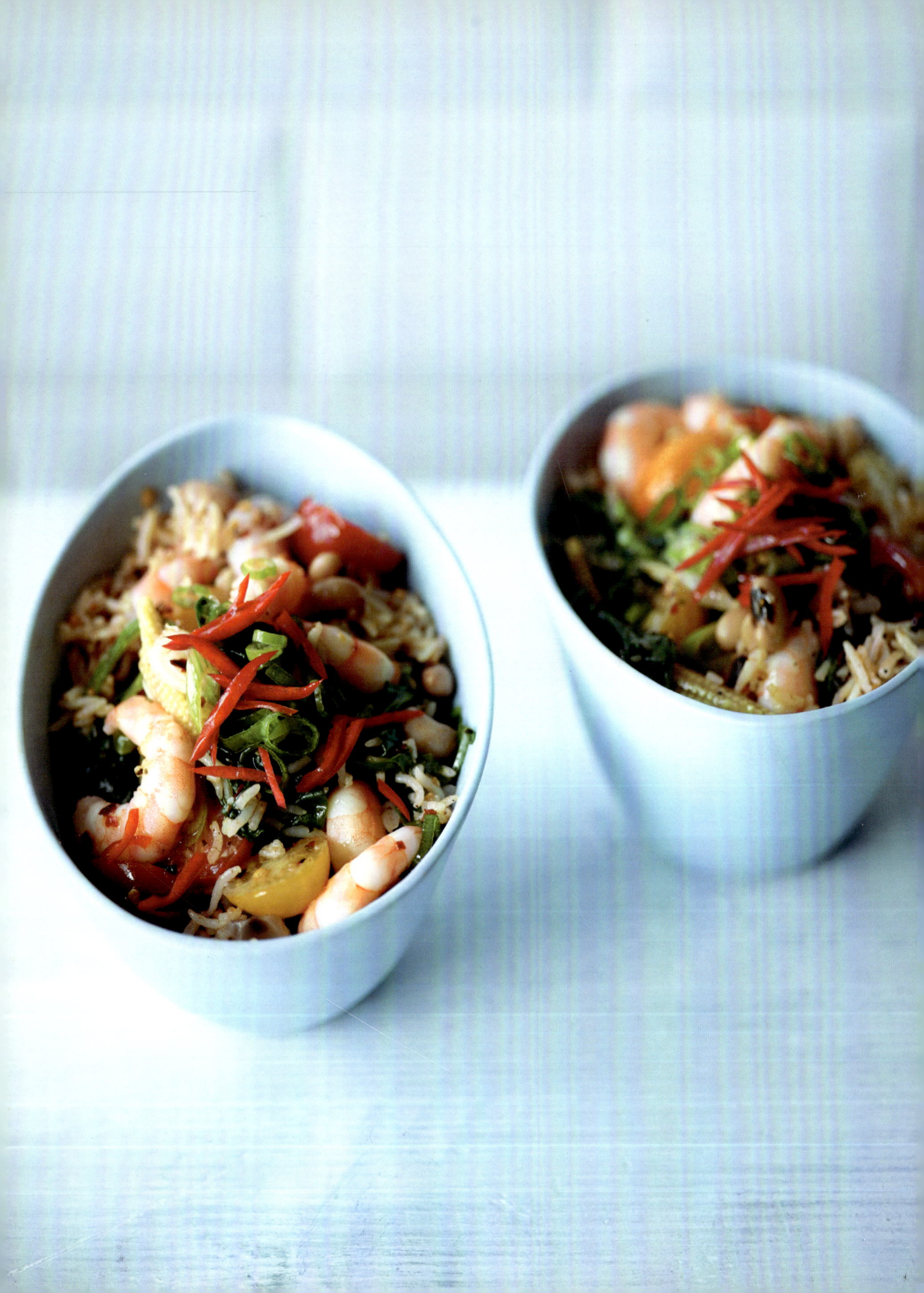

PIRI PIRI RICE WITH GARLIC PRAWNS

SERVES 1

I'm a massive fan of piri piri. It's one of my favourite seasonings and tastes awesome on most things. The black-eyed beans in this recipe add an extra protein boost. This is a great dish to double up, so you'll have some for lunch or dinner the next day.

MAKE AHEAD

INGREDIENTS

1 tbsp coconut oil
2 spring onions, roughly chopped
1 red chilli, roughly chopped – remove the seeds if you don't like it hot
6 baby sweetcorn, cut in half
4 cherry tomatoes, cut in half
2 tsp piri piri seasoning
100g tinned black-eyed beans, drained and rinsed
150g pre-cooked rice
large handful of baby spinach leaves
1 large clove garlic, chopped
12 raw prawns (about 200g), peeled
squeeze of lemon juice

METHOD

Heat half of the coconut oil in a wok or large frying pan over a high heat. Add the spring onions, chilli, sweetcorn and tomato and stir-fry for about 1 minute. Add the piri piri seasoning and stir-fry for 30 seconds, then add the black-eyed beans, along with 2 tablespoons of water. Add the rice, crumbling it between your fingers as you drop it in, then stir-fry for about 2 minutes, breaking up any clumps with a wooden spoon. Add the spinach, giving it a couple of turns to help it wilt. Tip the rice and vegetables onto a plate and wipe out your frying pan.

Return the wok or pan to a high heat and add the rest of the coconut oil. When it is melted and hot, add the garlic and prawns and cook for about 1 minute, stirring every now and then, until the prawns are pink and cooked through.

Spoon the garlicky prawns over the piri piri rice, finish with a squeeze of lemon juice and eat up.

SINGAPORE NOODLES

SERVES 1

When you finish a workout feeling ravenous, you want food, and you want it fast. This is the dish for such times. It might seem like a strange combination, but the chicken, curry powder and prawns are a total winner. If you don't fancy the combo, feel free to use either chicken or prawns – in which case, you'll need 250g chicken or 200g prawns.

MAKE AHEAD

INGREDIENTS

- 1 tbsp coconut oil
- 150g skinless chicken breast, sliced into 1cm thick strips
- 1 tbsp mild curry powder
- 8 prawns, peeled
- 2 spring onions, roughly chopped
- 1 red chilli, roughly chopped – remove the seeds if you don't like it hot
- 1 clove garlic, roughly chopped
- 50g mange tout, cut in half
- 6 baby sweetcorn, cut in half
- 200g fresh egg noodles
- salt and pepper
- juice of 1 lime
- ¼ bunch of coriander, leaves only, roughly chopped

METHOD

Heat the oil in a wok or large frying pan over a high heat. Add the chicken and fry for 1 minute, turning it a couple of times. When the chicken is no longer pink, sprinkle half of the curry powder into the wok and stir to coat the chicken strips.

Throw in the prawns and toss with the other ingredients. Add the spring onions, chilli, garlic, mange tout and sweetcorn and stir-fry for about 2 minutes or until the prawns are pink and the chicken is cooked through. Check the chicken by slicing into one of the larger pieces to make sure the meat is white all the way through, with no raw pink bits left.

Add the noodles, along with about 2 tablespoons of water – this will help to loosen any ingredients that may have stuck to the wok or pan, as well as helping to separate the noodles.

Sprinkle in the rest of the curry powder and season generously with salt and pepper. Toss everything together before piling the noodles onto a plate, drizzling over the lime juice and finishing with the chopped coriander.

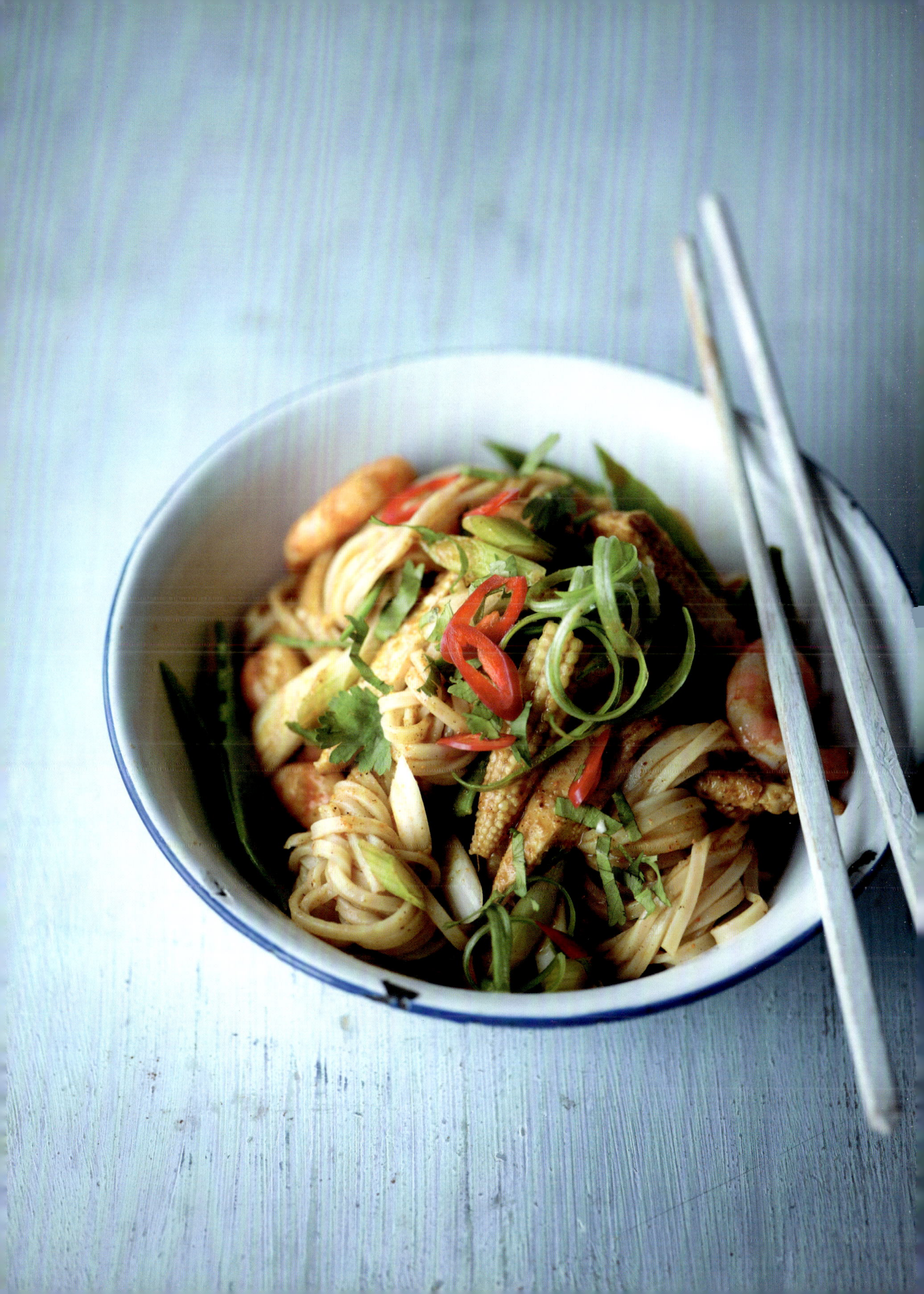

#BURGERME WITH SWEET POTATO FRIES

SERVES 2

I'm sorry but I refuse to release a cookbook without at least a couple of healthy burger recipes. Burgers make me happy, and I promise this one won't disappoint. Stack it up like a boss and get it done!

INGREDIENTS

- 2 large sweet potatoes, cut into fries
- 600g reduced-fat (about 5%) beef mince
- 1 small red onion, finely chopped
- 1 clove garlic, finely chopped
- salt and pepper
- 1 tbsp coconut oil
- 2 tsp chipotle paste
- 2 tbsp crème fraiche
- 2 burger buns
- 1 tomato, sliced
- 2 gherkins, sliced
- lettuce, to serve

METHOD

Preheat your grill to maximum.

Zap the sweet potato fries in the microwave for 7 minutes at 900w, then leave to rest for 30 seconds.

While the sweet potato is spinning in the microwave, mix the beef with the onion and garlic – get your hands stuck in and work the ingredients together with a good pinch each of salt and pepper. Shape the mixture into two good-sized burgers about 2cm thick. Place on your grill pan or a baking tray and grill for 5 minutes on each side.

Heat the coconut oil in a large frying pan over a high heat. Add the sweet potato fries and fry for about 3 minutes on each side or until they are nicely browned all over. Drain on paper towels, then season with a good pinch of salt.

Mix together the chipotle paste and crème fraiche in a small bowl.

Cut the burger buns in half, then build your burgers: start with a beef patty, then top with tomato, gherkins, lettuce and chipotle-crème fraiche sauce, finishing with the top half of the burger bun. Serve up with the sweet potato fries and shout out 'Hashtag BurgerMe' just before you eat it.

PRAWN, COURGETTE AND LENTIL CURRY

SERVES 1

We usually think it takes ages to cook a curry, but some can be lightning quick to make! You can use chicken instead of prawns if you want; even a bit of haddock would be good. And if you really want to mix it up, aubergine works as well as courgette, though you'll need to cook it for a bit longer. Don't be afraid to use ready-made curry pastes, either – they are lifesavers!

MAKE AHEAD
GOOD TO FREEZE

INGREDIENTS

- ½ tbsp coconut oil
- 1 small red onion, diced
- 1 courgette, diced
- 1 red chilli, sliced – optional
- 1 tbsp curry paste – I like Patak's rogan josh or bhuna
- 200g tinned chopped tomatoes
- 200g raw prawns, peeled
- 100g pre-cooked puy lentils
- 200g pre-cooked basmati rice
- ½ bunch of coriander, leaves only, roughly chopped

METHOD

Melt the coconut oil in a wok or large frying pan over a medium to high heat. Add the onion and courgette – and the chilli, if using – and stir-fry until starting to soften.

Spoon in the curry paste and fry for 30 seconds before pouring in the chopped tomatoes. Bring to the boil, then add the prawns and lentils. Simmer the curry for 1 minute or until the lentils are warmed through and the prawns are cooked – they're done when their flesh turns vibrant pink.

Meanwhile, ping your rice in the microwave, following the packet instructions.

Stir the coriander through your curry and serve up with the rice.

SERVES 1

MAKE AHEAD

MIGHTY DUCK NOODLES

It's good to switch up your bird now and again. This quick and easy duck noodle dish makes a nice change from your standard chicken and turkey. The five-spice and hoisin create an absolute explosion of flavour.

INGREDIENTS

- ½ tbsp coconut oil
- 1 x 240g duck breast fillet, skin removed, sliced into 1cm thick strips
- ½ tsp five-spice powder
- 3 spring onions, finely sliced
- 1 clove garlic, finely sliced
- 100g midget trees (tender-stem broccoli), any bigger stalks sliced in half lengthways
- 250g fresh egg noodles
- 2 tbsp hoisin sauce
- ¼ small cucumber, sliced into thin batons

METHOD

Melt the coconut oil in a wok or large frying pan over a medium to high heat. Add the duck and let it sizzle for a couple of minutes. When the duck is mostly brown, crank the heat up to high and add the five-spice powder, spring onions, garlic and midget trees, along with about 2 tablespoons of water – this will steam up and help everything to cook. Stir-fry for about 3 minutes, then add the noodles, and toss until the noodles are warmed through.

Remove from the heat and pour in the hoisin sauce. Stir everything together into one delicious mass, then slide onto a plate and top with the cucumber.

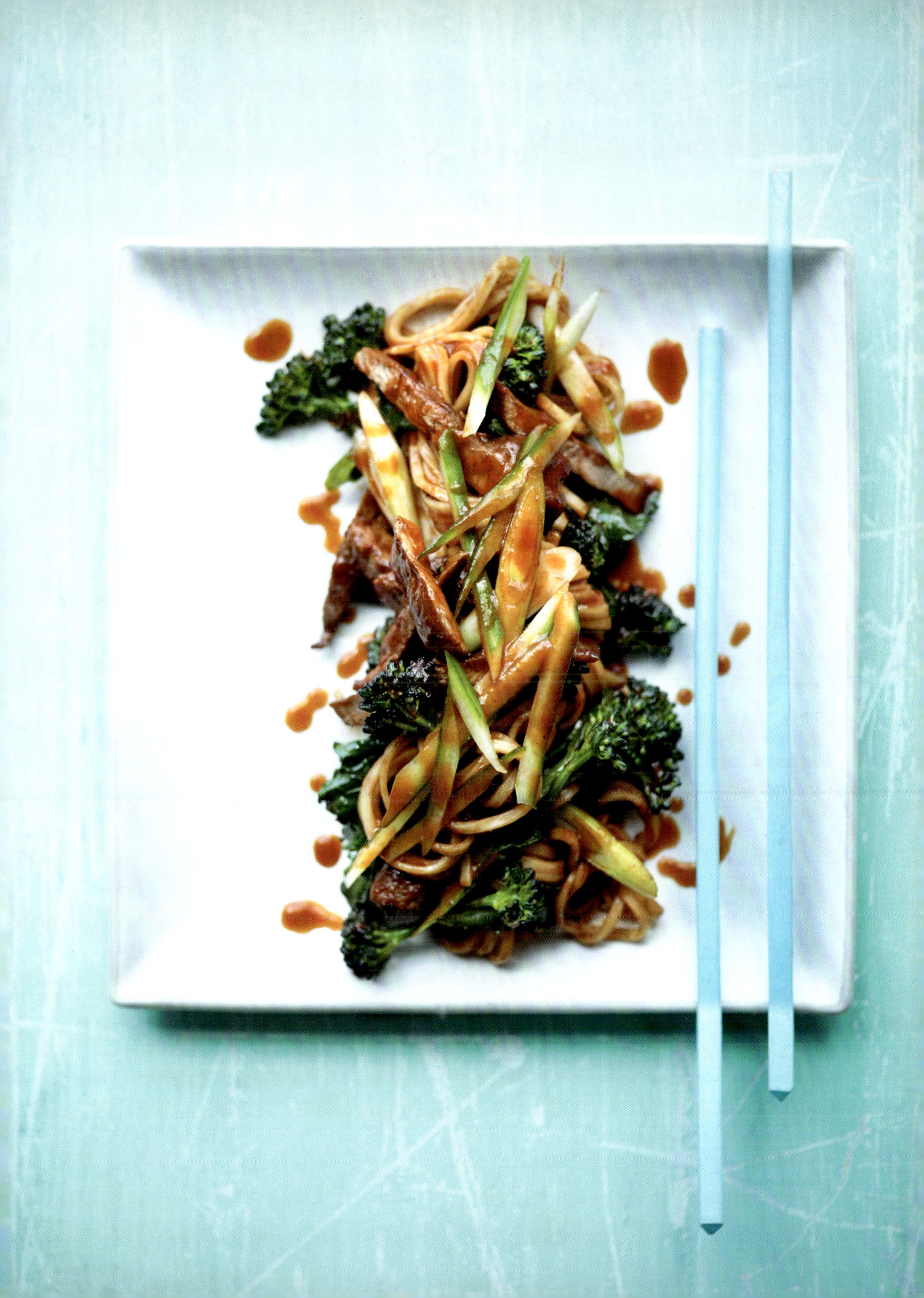

JOE'S McLEANIE BURGER

SERVES 2

Another burger recipe? Guilty. Well, I did say I love burgers. And remember a turkey is not just for Christmas – combined with all these tasty ingredients, you really won't be disappointed with this super-lean hero burger.

INGREDIENTS

400g turkey mince
3 tsp fish sauce
½ bunch of coriander, leaves only, roughly chopped
2 tsp sesame oil
4 spring onions, finely sliced
salt and pepper
2 burger buns
2 tbsp full-fat Greek yoghurt
3 tsp chipotle paste
sliced tomato and lettuce leaves, to serve

METHOD

Preheat your grill to its highest setting.

Chuck the turkey, fish sauce, coriander, sesame oil and spring onions into a large bowl. Season generously with salt and pepper, then get your hands stuck in and work the ingredients well. The more you work the meat, the better the burgers will hold together when cooked. Shape the meat into two equal patties.

Place the patties on your grill pan or a baking tray and grill the burgers for 5 minutes on each side or until they are totally cooked through. Check by slicing into one of the patties to make sure the meat is white all the way through, with no raw pink bits left.

Meanwhile, cut your burger buns in half. Mix together the yoghurt and chipotle paste and spread over the burger buns.

When your burgers are cooked, remove from the grill and build your dream burger, stacking it up with tomato and lettuce – the bigger, the better.

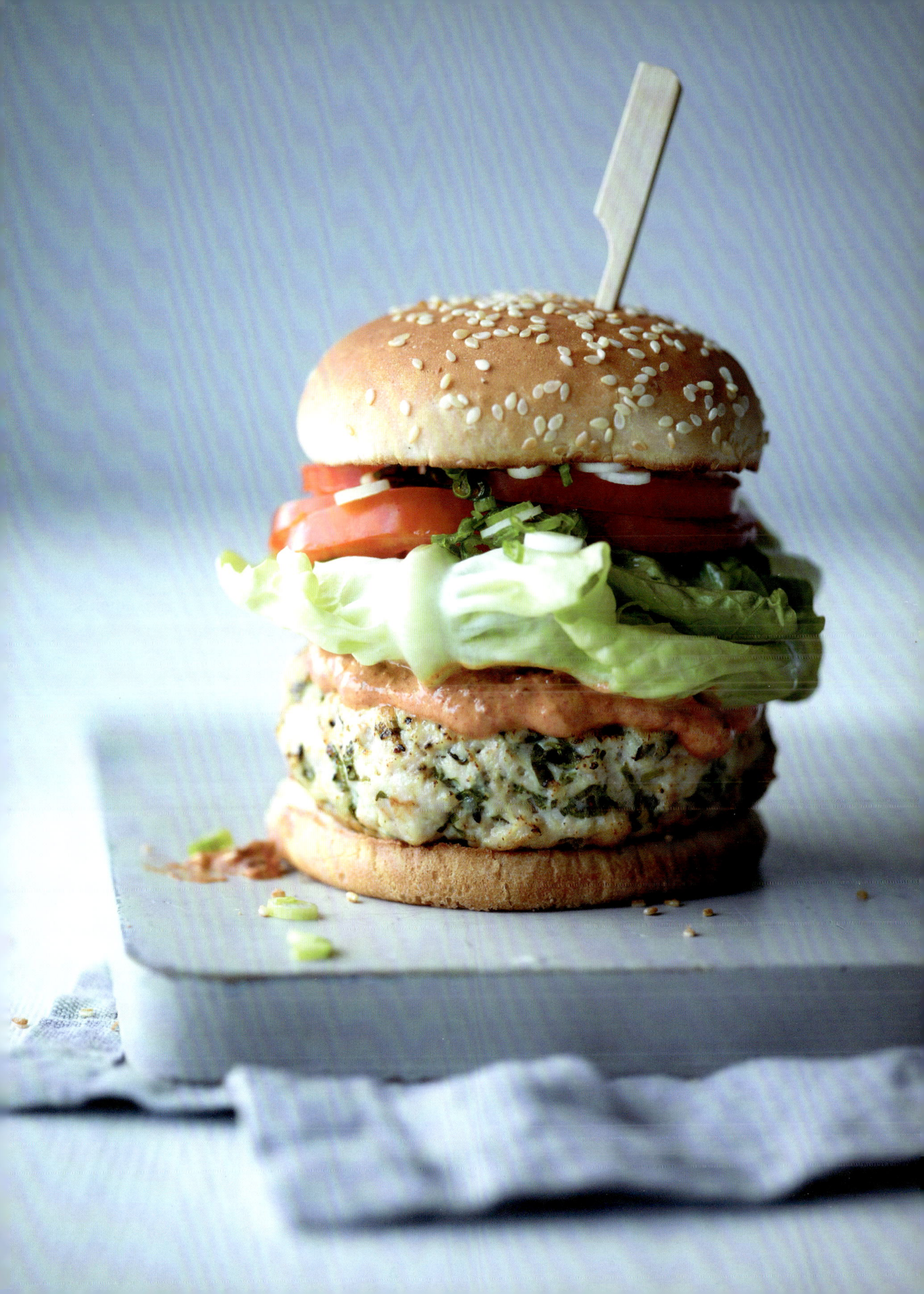

CHEEKY CHICKEN FRIED RICE

Do you ever just feel lazy and want to do as little work as possible in the kitchen? I do, and if you feel the same, then this one-wok, no-messing-about dish will be right up your street. Pre-cooked, packaged rice is a great thing to have in the house for a quick meal – and for this, it doesn't even have to go in the microwave. Almost any vegetables can go into this fried rice, making it a great way of using up the stragglers. It's perfect for lunch the next day too, so you can always do a cheeky double-up with the recipe. #Guilty

SERVES 1

MAKE AHEAD

INGREDIENTS

- 1 tbsp coconut oil
- 1 clove garlic, finely chopped
- 1cm ginger, finely chopped
- 1 x 240g skinless chicken breast fillet, sliced into 1cm thick strips
- 2 spring onions, roughly chopped
- 1 carrot, chopped into 1cm pieces
- 40g frozen peas
- 50g baby sweetcorn, roughly chopped
- 250g pre-cooked basmati rice
- 1 tbsp light soy sauce
- 2 tsp sesame oil
- ½ red chilli, finely chopped – optional

METHOD

Melt the coconut oil in a wok or large frying pan over a high heat. Throw in the garlic and ginger and stir-fry for 30 seconds.

Add the chicken and stir-fry for 2 minutes, by which time the chicken should have coloured a little on the outside. Chuck in the spring onions, carrot, peas and sweetcorn and stir-fry for another 2–3 minutes until the vegetables and chicken are cooked through. Check by slicing into one of the larger pieces of chicken to make sure the meat is white all the way through, with no raw pink bits left.

Tip in the rice straight from the packet, along with about 1 tablespoon of water, and keep stir-frying for about 1 minute or until the rice is warmed through.

Remove the wok or pan from the heat and pour in the soy sauce and sesame oil. Top with red chilli for added kick.

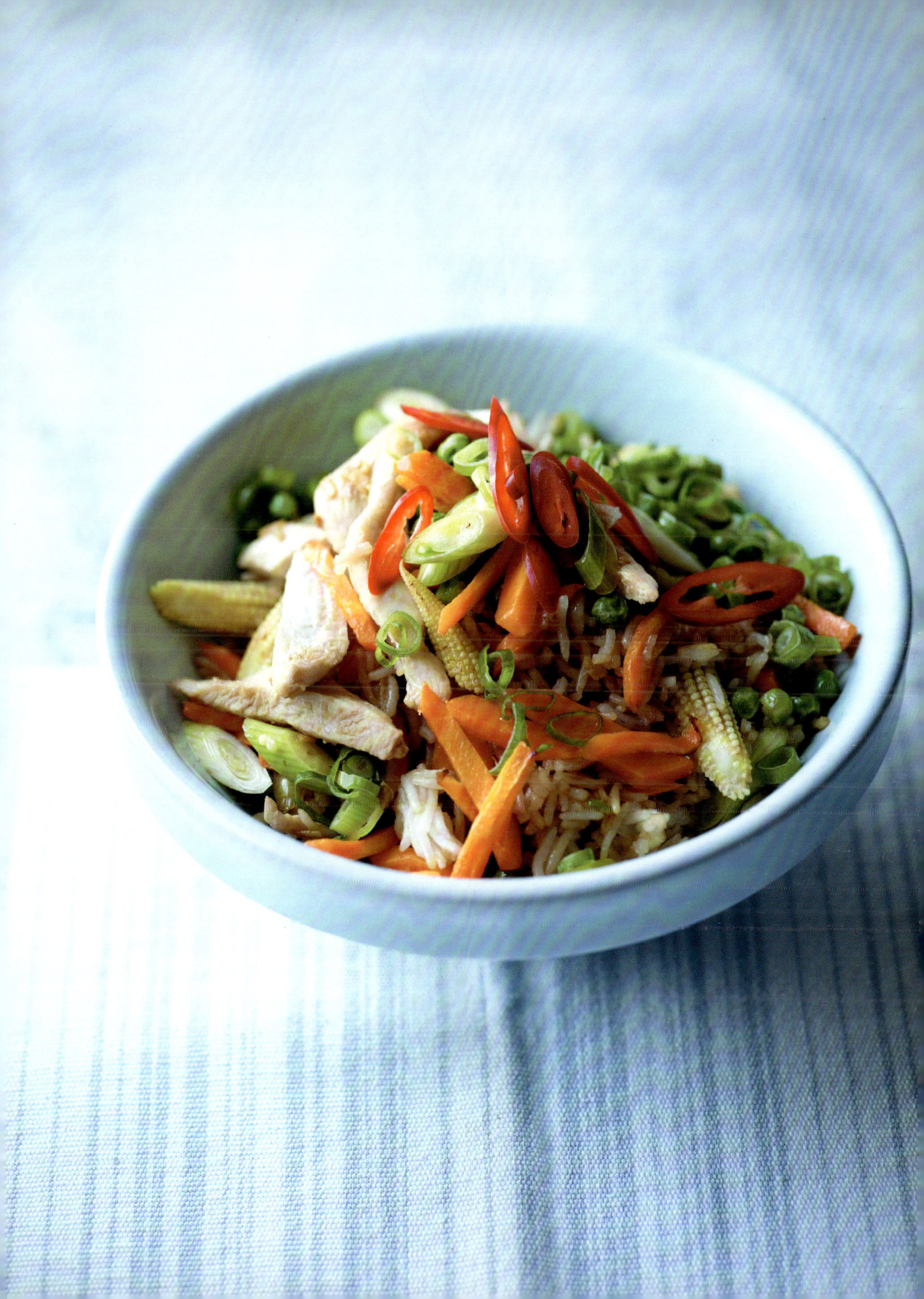

MY BIG JUICY MEATBALLS AND PASTA

SERVES 2

MAKE AHEAD
GOOD TO FREEZE
(only the meatballs, not the pasta)

INGREDIENTS

- 1 tbsp coconut oil
- 1 small red onion, diced
- 2 cloves garlic, finely chopped
- 2 sprigs of fresh thyme
- 1 x 400g tin of chopped tomatoes
- 12 (about 400g) ready-made turkey meatballs (or see page 93 to make your own)
- 2 large handfuls of baby spinach leaves
- salt and pepper
- 400g fresh tagliatelle
- ½ bunch of basil, leaves only, roughly chopped

Yes, that's right, pasta! Don't be scared – you can eat pasta and still burn fat. This food mountain will leave you feeling like a champion when you clear the plate. Fresh pasta cuts down the cooking time, but isn't essential. And if you can't find turkey meatballs, pork or beef meatballs work just as well.

METHOD

Start by bringing a large saucepan of water to the boil, ready to cook the pasta.

In a large frying pan or another large saucepan, heat the coconut oil over a medium to high heat. Add the onion, garlic and thyme to the pan and fry, stirring regularly, for 2 minutes or until the onion and garlic are just starting to soften. Pour in the tomatoes and bring to the boil. Carefully drop the meatballs into the sauce, then reduce the heat to a simmer and cover your pan with a lid. If you don't have a lid big enough, a large dinner plate or baking tray should do the trick. Simmer the meatballs for about 6 minutes, or until cooked through. Check by cutting into one to make sure there are no raw pink bits of meat left. Add the spinach to the sauce and stir until wilted. Season with salt and pepper, then remove the pan from the heat.

Drop the tagliatelle into the boiling water and cook for about 2 minutes. Drain the pasta and tip it back into the pan. Spoon in about half of the meatballs and sauce and mix with the pasta. Divide the saucy pasta between two plates, spoon over the remaining sauce and garnish with the basil.

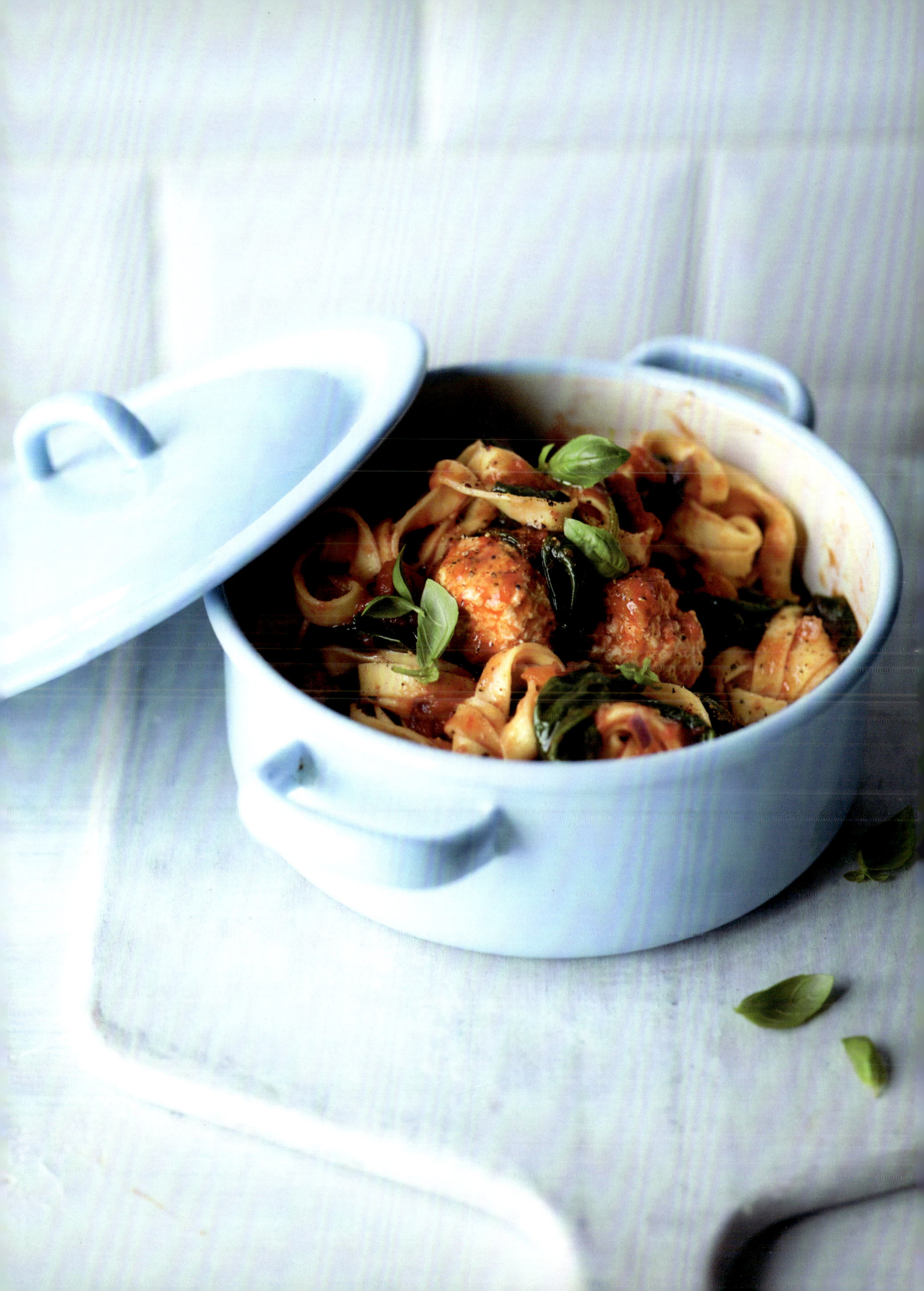

SERVES 1

KEDGEREE

This kedgeree (#weirdwordalert) tastes incredible – after a workout, it will refuel your body and satisfy your taste buds at the same time.

MAKE AHEAD
GOOD TO FREEZE

INGREDIENTS

½ tbsp coconut oil
2 spring onions, finely sliced
275g smoked haddock, skinned and cut into small chunks
1 courgette, cut into 2cm cubes
100g frozen peas
1 tbsp mild curry powder
1 egg
250g pre-cooked basmati rice
100ml skimmed milk
large handful of baby spinach leaves
1 red chilli, finely sliced – remove the seeds if you don't like it hot

METHOD

Bring a saucepan of water to the boil, ready to poach the egg.

Melt the coconut oil in a large frying pan over a medium to high heat. Add the spring onions, smoked haddock and courgette and fry for 2–3 minutes, stirring regularly. Stir in the peas and cook until defrosted, then sprinkle in the curry powder and cook for 1 minute.

This is a good time to carefully crack your egg into the hot water to poach. Cook the egg for about 4 minutes for a runny yolk, then carefully lift out with a slotted spoon and drain on paper towels.

While the egg is poaching, add the rice to the frying pan, crumbling it between your fingers as you drop it in, then stir-fry for a minute or two, breaking up any clumps with a wooden spoon. Pour in the milk and stir, then bring to the boil and simmer for about 30 seconds. Add the spinach and stir until wilted.

Pile the kedgeree onto a plate, top with the poached egg and scatter with sliced chilli, then serve.

SERVES 2

GNOCCHI WITH SAUSAGE RAGU

This little Italian number is guaranteed to please. The gnocchi cooks in no time, and the sausages are already full of flavour, making this a really tasty meal for very little effort.

MAKE AHEAD

GOOD TO FREEZE

INGREDIENTS

1 tbsp olive oil
1 red onion, diced
1 clove garlic, chopped
1 sprig of rosemary
6 sausages
1 tbsp balsamic vinegar
1 x 400g tin of chopped tomatoes
300g fresh gnocchi
½ bunch basil, leaves only, roughly chopped

METHOD

Bring a large saucepan of water to the boil, ready to cook the gnocchi.

In a frying pan, heat the olive oil over a medium to high heat. Add the onion, garlic and rosemary and cook, stirring occasionally, for 2–3 minutes.

Taking one sausage at a time, squeeze tightly with your fingers about a third of the way along its length to force the meat from the sausage skin – a small ball of sausage meat should pop out of the end of the casing. Repeat the process until you have 18 balls of sausage meat. Discard the empty sausage skins.

Drop the balls of sausage meat into the frying pan, and gently tumble them around the pan to coat in the oil, onion and garlic. Crank up the heat to high and pour in the balsamic vinegar, then let it bubble away to almost nothing. Pour in the tomatoes, bring to the boil and simmer for 5–6 minutes.

Meanwhile, drop the gnocchi into the pan of boiling water and cook for about 2 minutes, or according to the packet instructions, then drain.

Check that the balls of sausage meat are fully cooked through – cut into one to make sure – then divvy up the gnocchi, top with the sausage ragu and finish with the basil.

SAMMY THE SEA BASS WITH SPAGHETTI

SERVES 1

You may notice on Instagram that I like to name my foods – and somehow Sammy the Sea Bass seems to fit this dish. You won't believe how easy this one is. The other great thing is that you can add any leftover veg from the fridge as well . . . But please don't forget to shout, 'Bosh, midget trees' when you throw the broccoli in the pan!

INGREDIENTS

- 80g dried spaghetti
- ½ tbsp olive oil
- 2 x 125g sea bass fillets, skin on
- salt and pepper
- 80g midget trees (tender-stem broccoli), any bigger stalks sliced in half lengthways
- 80g kale, thick stalks removed
- 6 cherry tomatoes
- ½ red chilli, roughly sliced – remove the seeds if you don't like it hot

METHOD

Bring a large saucepan of salted water to the boil. Drop in the spaghetti and let it cook for 2 minutes less than the time given on the packet.

Meanwhile, heat the oil in a frying pan over a medium heat. Season the sea bass with salt and pepper, and when the oil is hot, gently lay the fillets in the pan, skin side down, and fry for 2–3 minutes. Flip the fish over, remove the pan from the heat and leave the fish to cook in the residual heat for 2 minutes. Carefully lift the fish out of the pan, then peel off and discard the skin.

By now the spaghetti should be almost cooked. Throw in all of the veg, and simmer with the pasta for 2 minutes. The tomatoes may split a little, but don't worry. Drain the pasta and veg in a colander.

Take the pan used to fry the fish and place it back over a medium to high heat. Tip in the spaghetti and veg, season generously with salt and pepper, and toss everything together for 1 minute – this final frying gives the dish extra flavour.

Spoon the spaghetti and vegetables into a shallow bowl, flake over the fish in large chunks and top with the sliced chilli.

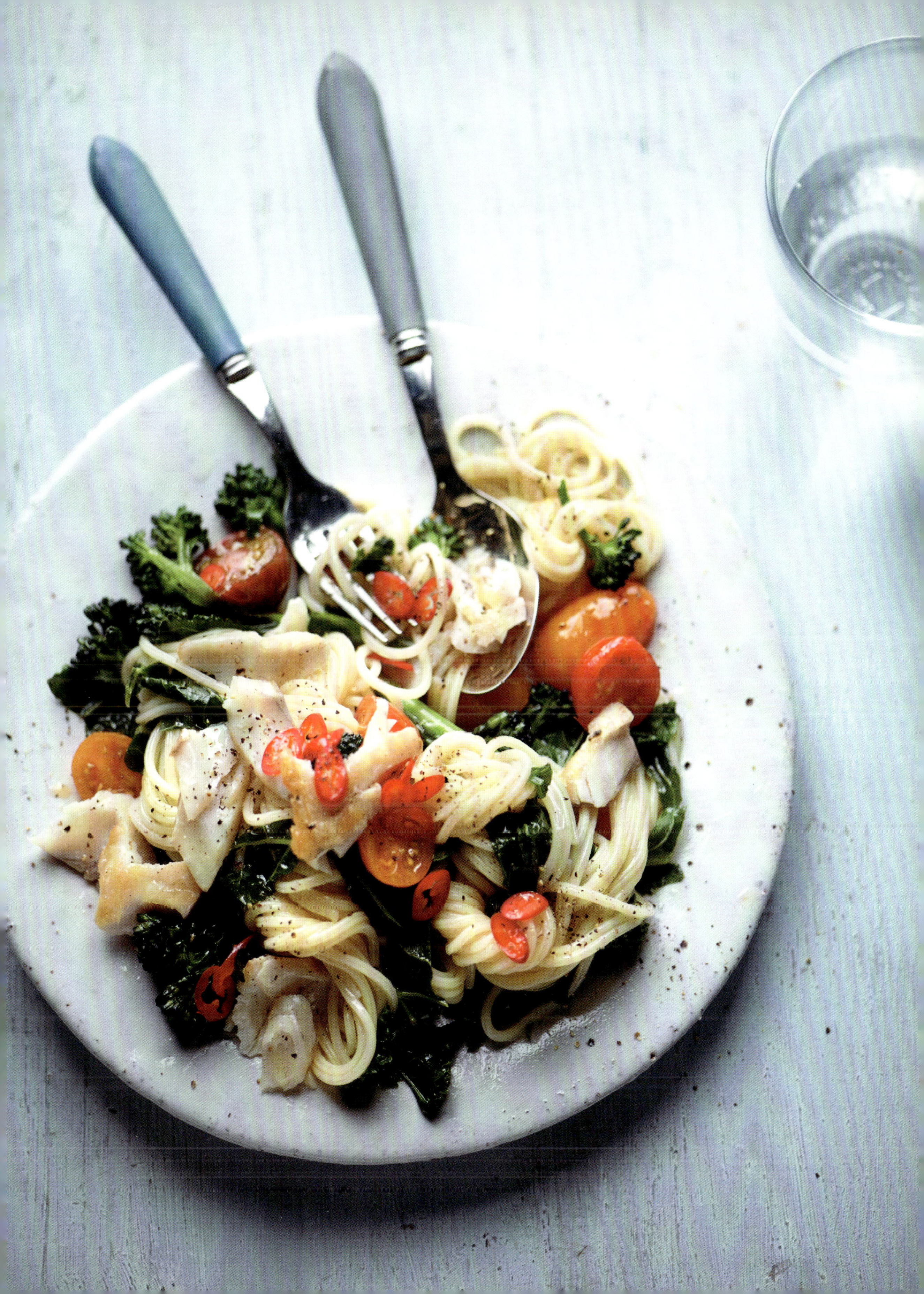

CHICKEN AND QUINOA STIR-FRY

SERVES 1

Quinoa used to be one of those obscure health foods, but these days it's everywhere – and luckily you can now get it pre-cooked in packets, so you don't have to wait 20 minutes for it to cook. The high protein content of quinoa makes this a great meal for building lean muscle.

MAKE AHEAD

INGREDIENTS

- ½ tbsp coconut oil
- 3 spring onions, finely sliced
- ½ red pepper, de-seeded and finely diced
- ½ courgette, diced
- 1 x 240g skinless chicken breast fillet, cut into 1cm thick slices
- 2 tsp smoked paprika
- salt and pepper
- 225g pre-cooked quinoa
- 25g feta, crumbled
- small bunch of parsley, leaves only, roughly chopped – optional
- squeeze of lemon juice

METHOD

Melt the coconut oil in a wok or large frying pan over a medium to high heat. Add the spring onions, red pepper and courgette and stir-fry for 2–3 minutes or until the vegetables are just starting to soften.

Increase the heat to high and add the chicken, along with the paprika and a little salt and pepper. Fry for a further 3–4 minutes or until the chicken is just cooked. Check by slicing into one of the larger pieces to make sure the meat is white all the way through, with no raw pink bits left.

Stir in the quinoa and fry for a minute or so, until it is warmed through.

Serve your chicken and quinoa stir-fry topped with crumbled feta, chopped parsley (if using) and a squeeze of lemon juice.

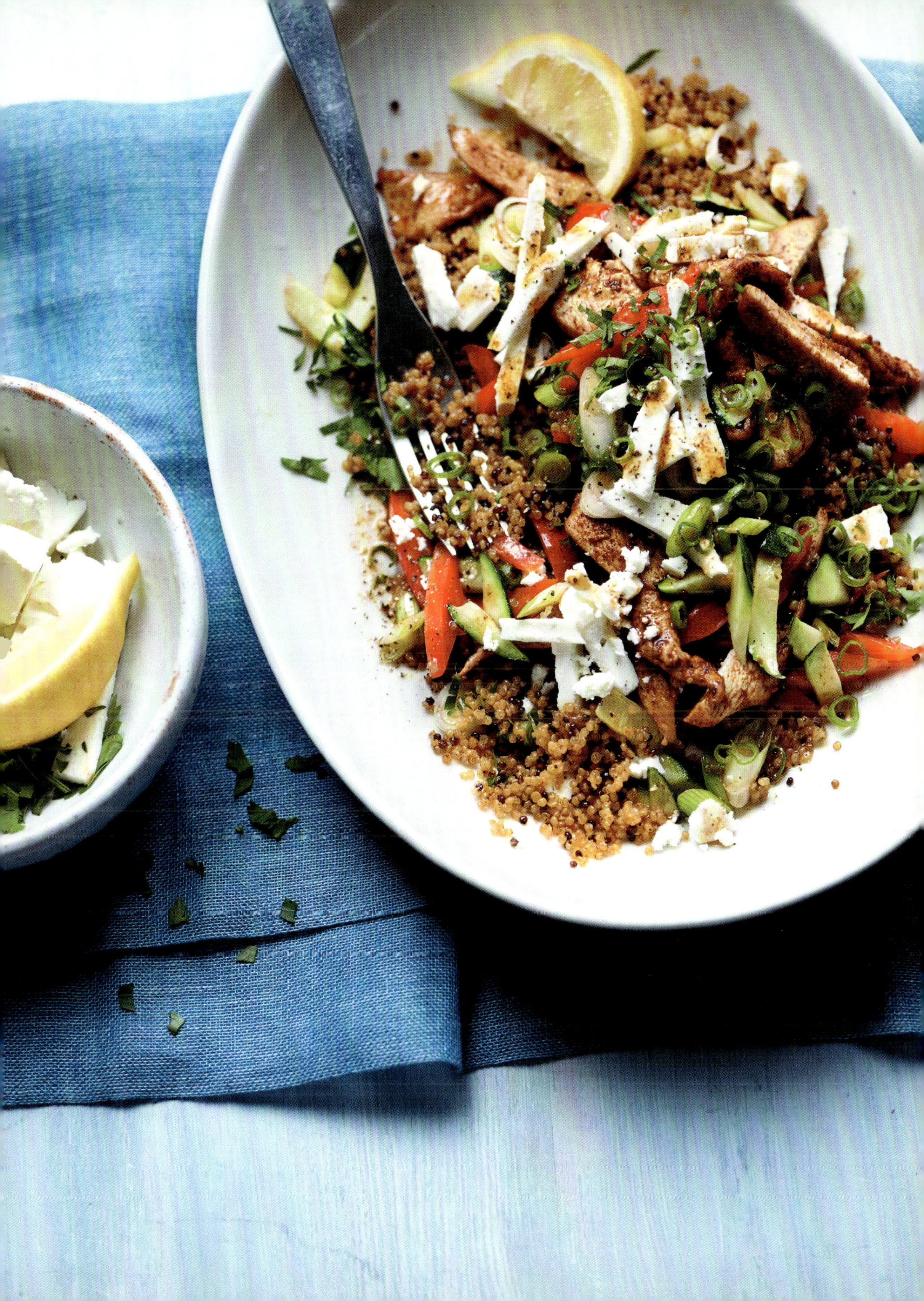

QUICK TORTILLA PIZZA

SERVES 1

This recipe is for all the pizza lovers out there. It may not have exactly the same effect as a cheesy stuffed-crust pizza, but it's cheaper, quicker and much leaner. Feel free to change the toppings and build your own dream pizza.

INGREDIENTS

- 4 large handfuls of baby spinach leaves
- 2 large tortillas
- 200g tinned chopped tomatoes
- 200g tinned kidney beans, rinsed and drained
- ½ tsp dried oregano
- 8 black olives, pitted and cut in half
- 250g sliced cooked meat – I like ham or cold roast chicken
- 2 large eggs
- salt and pepper
- green salad, to serve – optional

METHOD

Put the kettle on to boil and preheat your oven to 230°C (fan 210°C, gas mark 8).

Tip the spinach into a large colander and pour over boiling water from the kettle until it wilts. Quickly run the spinach under cold water to cool, then use your hands to squeeze out as much moisture as possible.

Place the tortillas on a non-stick baking tray. Mix together the tomatoes, kidney beans and oregano, then spread over the tortillas. Divide the wilted spinach evenly between the tortillas, then scatter over the olives and meat. Make a little well in the middle of each tortilla pizza and crack in an egg. Season the pizzas with salt and pepper, then slip into the hot oven and bake for 12 minutes, or until the edges are browned and the white of the egg is set.

Slide the pizzas onto a board and serve with a big green salad . . . or just wolf down.

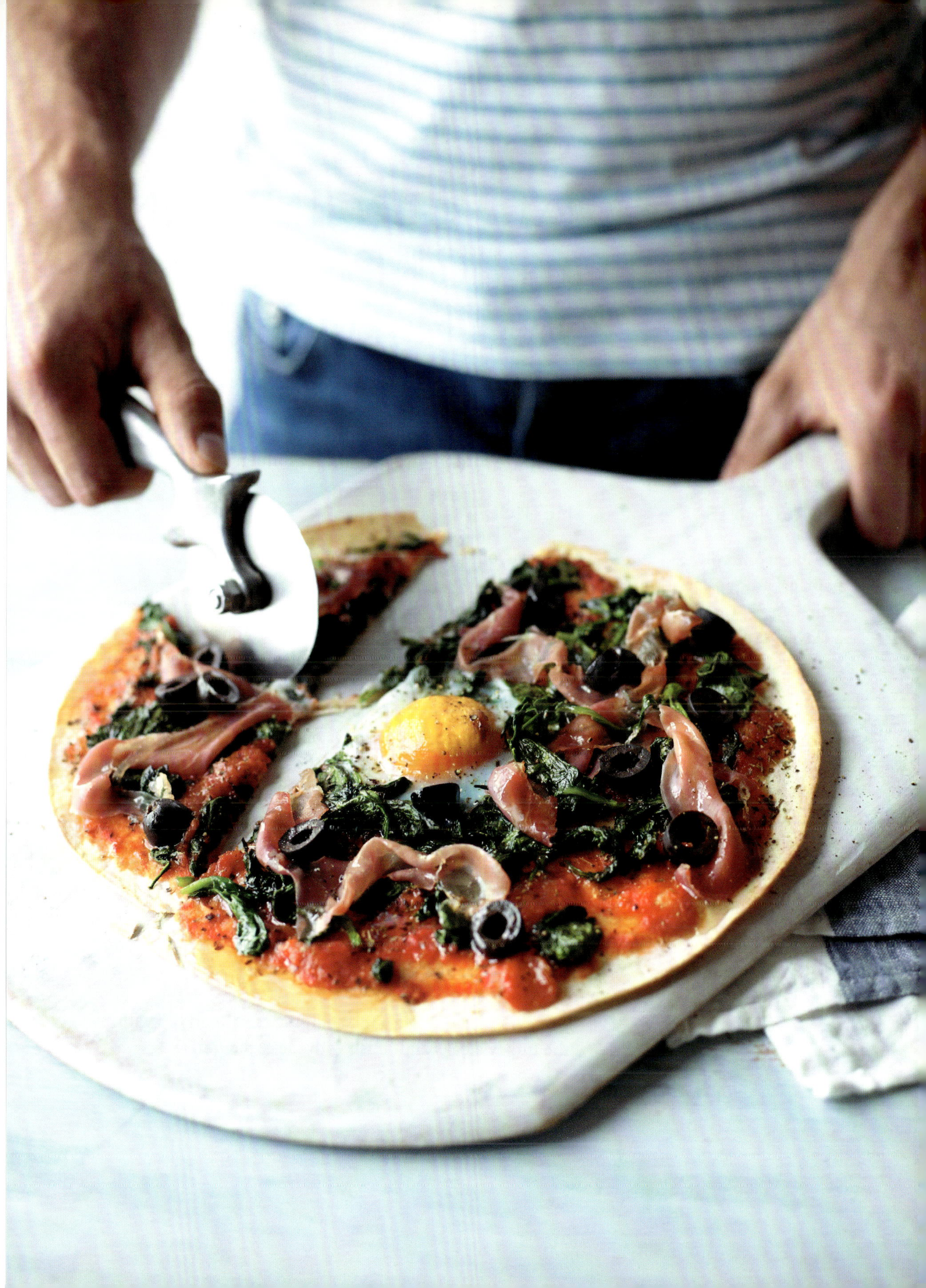

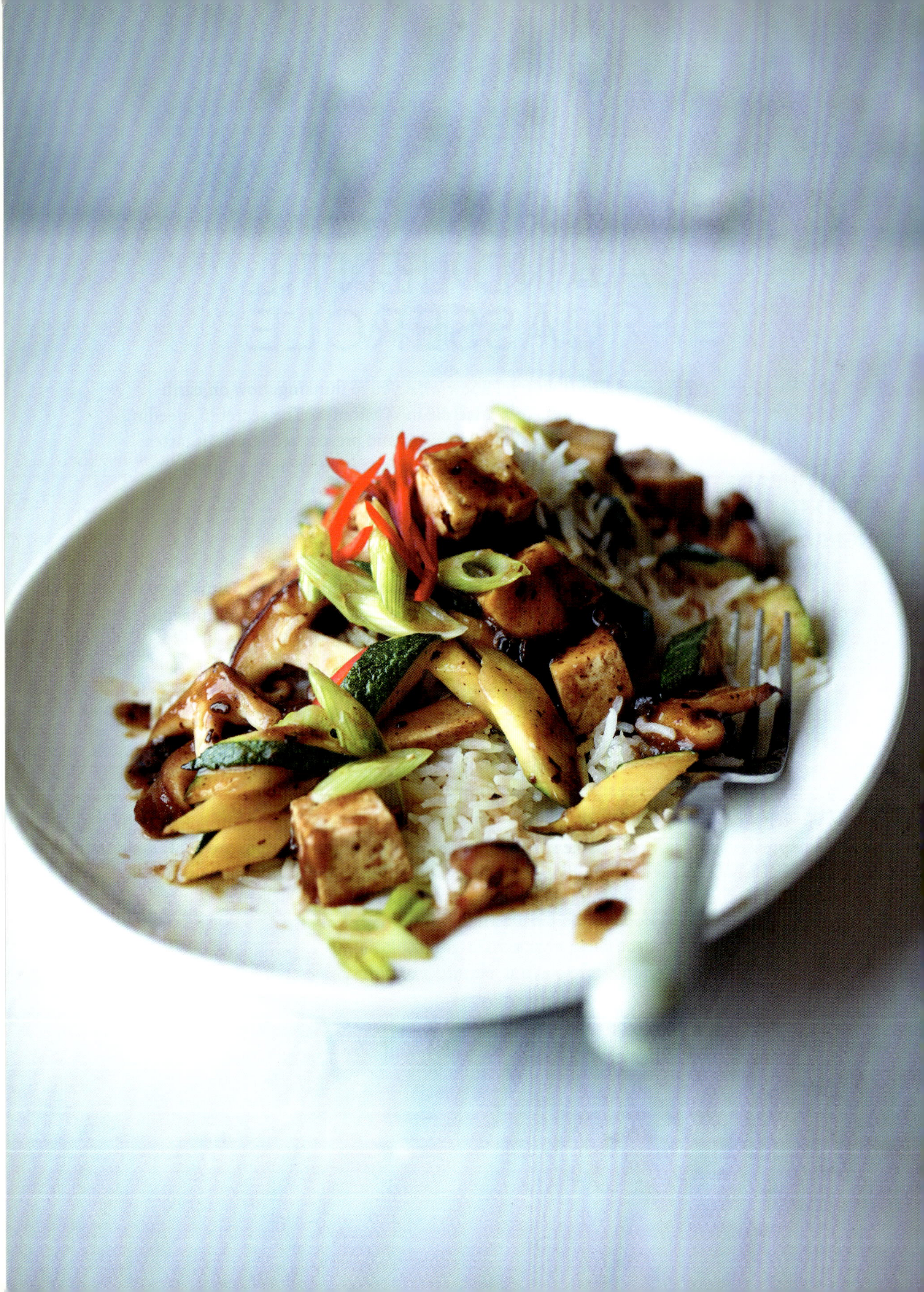

BLACK BEAN TOFU WITH SHIITAKE AND RICE

SERVES 2

I do apologize for the lack of veggie recipes, but I'm a meat-lover myself! Here's one that vegetarians, meat eaters and pescatarians will all love, though. When cooked with the right ingredients and flavours, tofu is really tasty – and if you eat a big enough portion, you can get a decent protein hit.

MAKE AHEAD

INGREDIENTS

1 tbsp coconut oil
1 courgette, cut into 1cm dice
1 red chilli, roughly chopped – remove the seeds if you don't like it hot
2 cloves garlic, roughly chopped
6 spring onions, cut into 1cm slices
8 shiitake mushrooms, roughly chopped
2 tbsp black bean sauce
400g firm tofu, cut into 2cm cubes
250g pre-cooked jasmine or basmati rice

METHOD

Heat the coconut oil in a wok or large frying pan over a medium to high heat. Throw in the courgette and stir-fry for 1 minute. Add the chilli, garlic, spring onions and shiitake and stir-fry for 3–4 minutes, or until all the vegetables are starting to soften.

Spoon in the black bean sauce and pour in 150ml of water. Bring to a simmer, then drop in the tofu and simmer gently for about 2 minutes or until heated through.

Ping your rice in the microwave and divide it between two plates, then top with the spicy, rich tofu.

TERIYAKI CHICKEN STIR-FRY

SERVES 1

This is one of those dishes you'll love so much you'll want to make it every day. You can just walk in from work and smash this all in a wok, with little mess to clear up afterwards – a true Lean in 15 recipe.

MAKE AHEAD

INGREDIENTS

- ½ tbsp coconut oil
- 3 spring onions, finely sliced
- 2 cloves garlic, finely sliced
- 2cm ginger, finely chopped or grated
- 1 x 240g skinless chicken breast fillet, sliced into 1 cm thick strips
- 2 heads of pak choy, leaves separated
- 225g fresh egg noodles
- large handful of baby spinach leaves
- ½ tbsp honey
- 1 tbsp light soy sauce
- 2 tsp rice wine vinegar
- 1 red chilli, finely sliced – remove the seeds if you don't like it hot

METHOD

Heat the coconut oil in a wok or large frying pan over a high heat. Add the spring onions, garlic and ginger and stir-fry for 10 seconds, then add the chicken and stir-fry for 1 minute.

Throw in the pak choy, noodles, spinach and a couple of tablespoons of water – this will create steam to help cook the vegetables and separate the noodles. Stir-fry for 2–3 minutes, by which time the vegetables will have wilted and the chicken should be totally cooked through. Check by slicing into one of the larger pieces to make sure the meat is white all the way through, with no raw pink bits left.

Remove from the heat and pour in the honey, soy sauce and vinegar, mixing well. Pile the stir-fry onto a plate, top with the sliced chilli and get it down you.

★ TOP TIP

If you can't find fresh egg noodles, just use dried ones – but remember they'll need rehydrating before you add them to the stir-fry. And for a gluten-free meal, swap the soy sauce for tamari, and use rice noodles instead of egg noodles.

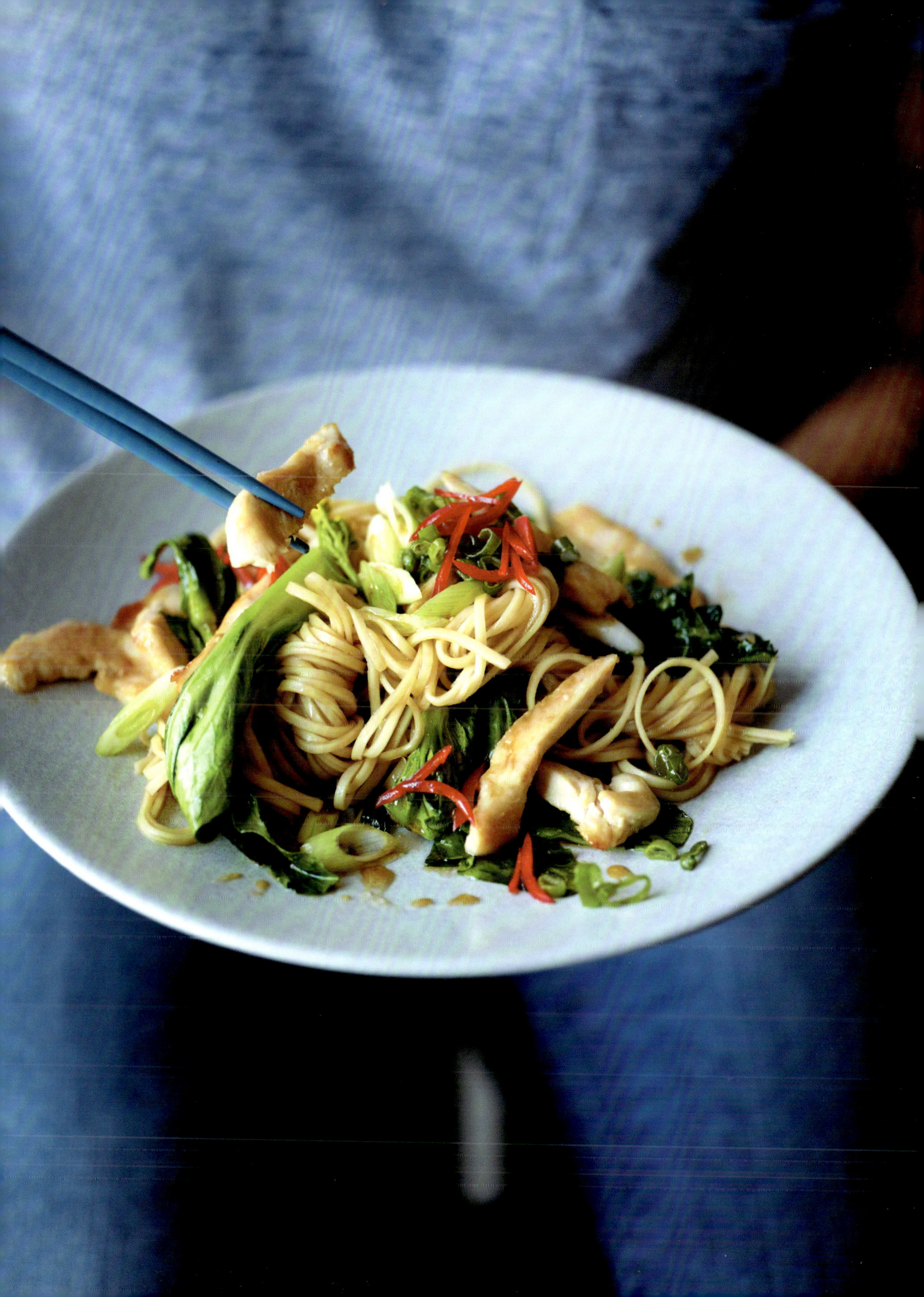

BIG BARBECUE CHICKEN WRAP

SERVES 1

This easy chicken wrap with barbecue sauce goes down a treat after a workout. Wrapped up tightly in foil, it's the ideal lunch on the go.

MAKE AHEAD

INGREDIENTS

- 1 x 240g skinless chicken breast fillet
- salt and pepper
- 1 tbsp tomato ketchup
- ½ tsp smoked paprika
- 1 tbsp Worcestershire sauce
- 2 large tortilla wraps
- 1 baby gem lettuce, shredded
- 6 cherry tomatoes, halved
- 4 tbsp tinned black-eyed beans, drained and rinsed
- 2 tbsp cottage cheese

METHOD

Preheat your grill to maximum.

Spread out a large piece of cling film on your chopping board or benchtop. Lay the chicken on the cling film and place another piece of cling film on top. Using a rolling pin, heavy saucepan or any other blunt object, bash the chicken until it is at least half its original thickness.

Remove the chicken from the cling film and season with salt and pepper, then place on your grill pan or a baking tray and grill for 4 minutes, without turning.

Meanwhile, mix together the ketchup, paprika and Worcestershire sauce until you have a smooth barbecue sauce. Flip the chicken over and give it 2 more minutes, then smear over a little of the sauce and grill for a further 3–4 minutes, or until it is fully cooked through. Check by slicing into it to make sure the meat is white all the way through, with no raw pink bits left.

Slice the cooked chicken into long strips. Spread the remaining barbecue sauce over the tortillas, then top with the chicken, lettuce, tomatoes, beans and cottage cheese. Roll up your big fat tortillas and get munching.

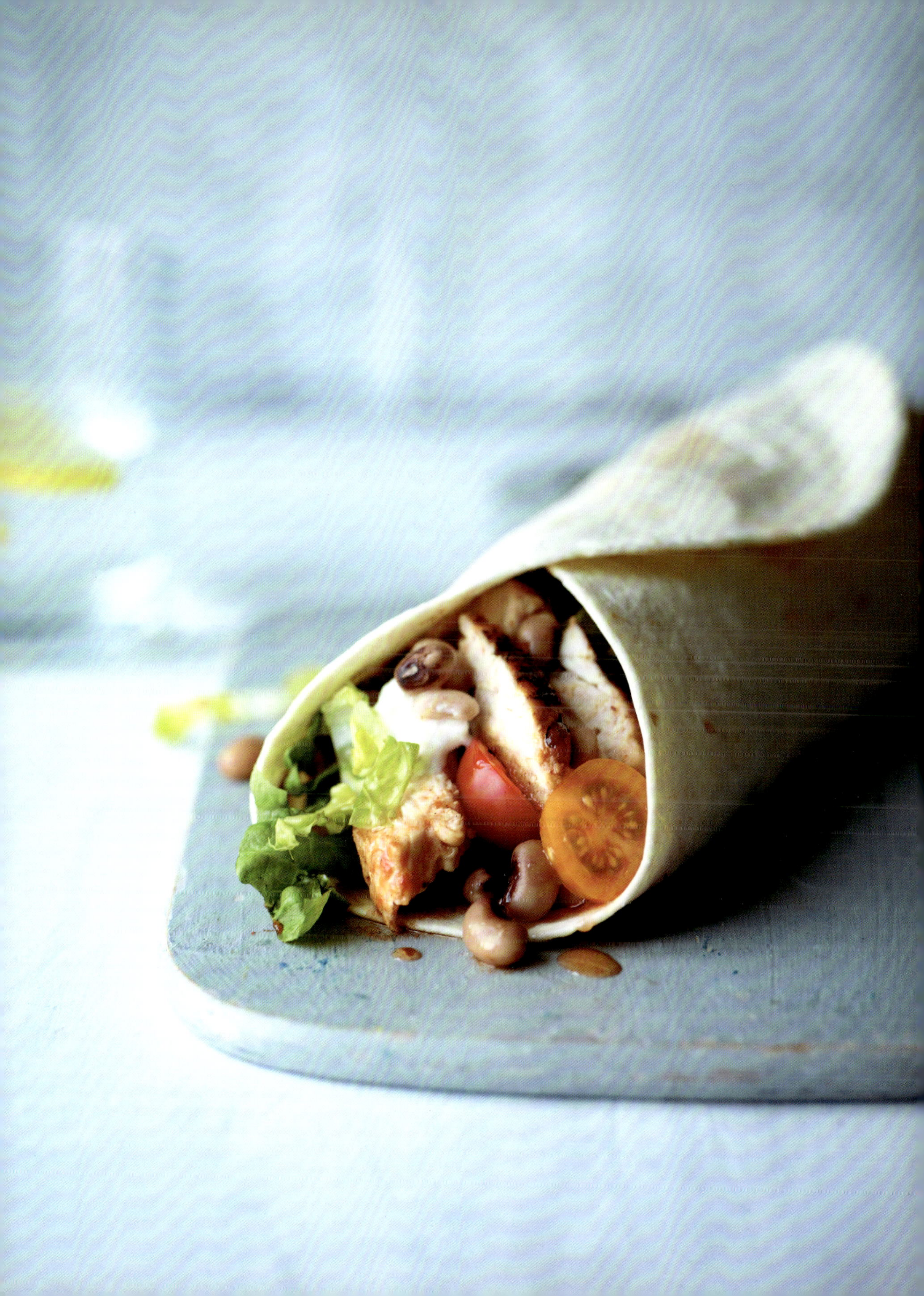

TOMATO DAAL WITH CHICKEN

SERVES 2

LONGER RECIPE
MAKE AHEAD
GOOD TO FREEZE

INGREDIENTS

150g yellow split peas
1½ tbsp coconut oil
1 tsp cumin seeds
1 fresh bay leaf, or 2 dried
1 large red onion, diced
4 cloves garlic, finely chopped
2 red chillies, diced – remove the seeds if you don't like it hot
5cm ginger, diced
½ tsp ground turmeric
1 tbsp garam masala
5 large tomatoes, roughly chopped
200–250ml chicken stock
2 x 260g skinless chicken breast fillets, sliced into 1cm strips
salt and pepper
bunch of coriander, leaves only, roughly chopped

Clocking in at about an hour, this is another recipe that takes longer than 15 minutes. Don't be put off, though – it's full of flavour and really satisfying after a workout, so it's worth the wait. If you're after a short cut, batch-cook the daal and freeze the extra, ready for the next time.

METHOD

Tip the split peas into a large bowl and cover with warm water from the tap, then leave to soak for at least 20 minutes.

Melt 1 tablespoon of the coconut oil in a large saucepan over a medium to high heat. Add the cumin seeds and bay leaf and fry for 30 seconds, then add the onion and stir-fry for 2–3 minutes or until just starting to soften and brown. Drop in the garlic, chillies and ginger and stir-fry for 1 minute.

Sprinkle in the turmeric and the garam masala and stir constantly for 30 seconds. Chuck in the tomatoes and chicken stock, then bring to the boil. Drain and rinse the soaked split peas and add them to the pan. Simmer for about 40 minutes, stirring regularly, and adding a little extra water if necessary, by which time the split peas should be completely cooked and starting to fall apart.

When the daal is nearly ready, melt the remaining coconut oil in a frying pan and add the chicken, seasoning it generously with salt and pepper. Fry for about 3 minutes or until the chicken is cooked through. Check by slicing into one of the larger pieces to make sure the meat is white all the way through, with no raw pink bits left.

Stir the coriander through the cooked daal, top with the chicken and serve.

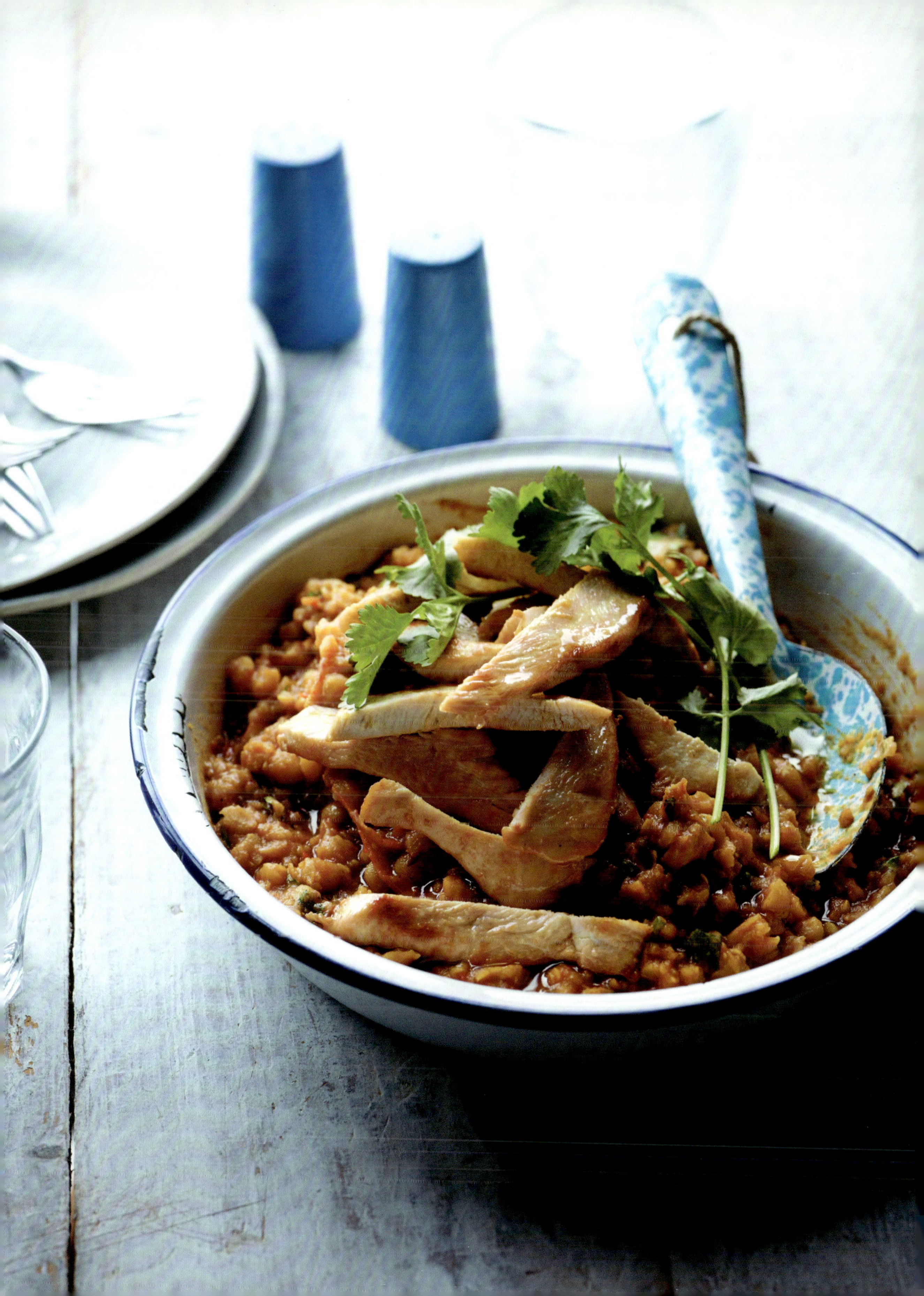

MY MUM'S SPECIAL LASAGNE

SERVES 4

LONGER RECIPE
MAKE AHEAD
GOOD TO FREEZE

INGREDIENTS

- 1½ tbsp olive oil
- 1kg reduced-fat (about 5%) beef mince
- 1 large red onion, diced
- 1 carrot, diced
- 1 courgette, diced
- 2 cloves garlic, finely chopped
- 1 tbsp tomato puree
- 400ml beef stock
- 1 x 400g tin of chopped tomatoes
- 18 lasagne sheets
- bunch of basil, leaves only, roughly torn – optional
- crusty bread, to serve

This is my mum's special recipe. In fact, as she would say, it's the only thing she can cook. She's Italian, and when she was growing up, she used to make this almost every week. Being a lasagne, it takes more like an hour and 15 minutes from start to finish, but it doesn't take too long to prep – and once it's in the oven you can sit back and relax. I'm sure you will love this, just like I always have.

METHOD

Heat ½ tablespoon of the olive oil in a large saucepan over a high heat. Add half the mince and fry for 2–3 minutes, stirring to break up the chunks. Tip out onto a plate, then repeat with another ½ tablespoon of oil and the rest of the mince.

When the meat has all been browned, wipe out your pan and heat the remaining ½ tablespoon of oil over a medium to high heat. Add the onion, carrot, courgette and garlic and cook, stirring regularly, for about 5 minutes – by which time the vegetables should have started to soften and colour a little. Add the tomato puree, beef stock and tomatoes, then return the mince to the pan. Bring to a simmer and cook for 20 minutes.

Preheat the oven to 190°C (fan 170°C, gas mark 5).

Start building your lasagne in a baking dish about 30cm x 15cm. Spoon in about a quarter of the meat sauce, spreading it over the base of the dish, then lay 6 sheets of pasta on top (don't worry too much if they overlap). Repeat the process until you have four layers of meat sauce and three layers of pasta – your last layer should be a layer of meat sauce. Tightly cover the dish with foil and bake in the oven for 40 minutes, or until it is heated through and the pasta is fully cooked – you should be able to easily insert a fork into the lasagne.

Finish the lasagne with a scattering of freshly torn basil, if you like, and serve with a chunk of bread and a green salad.

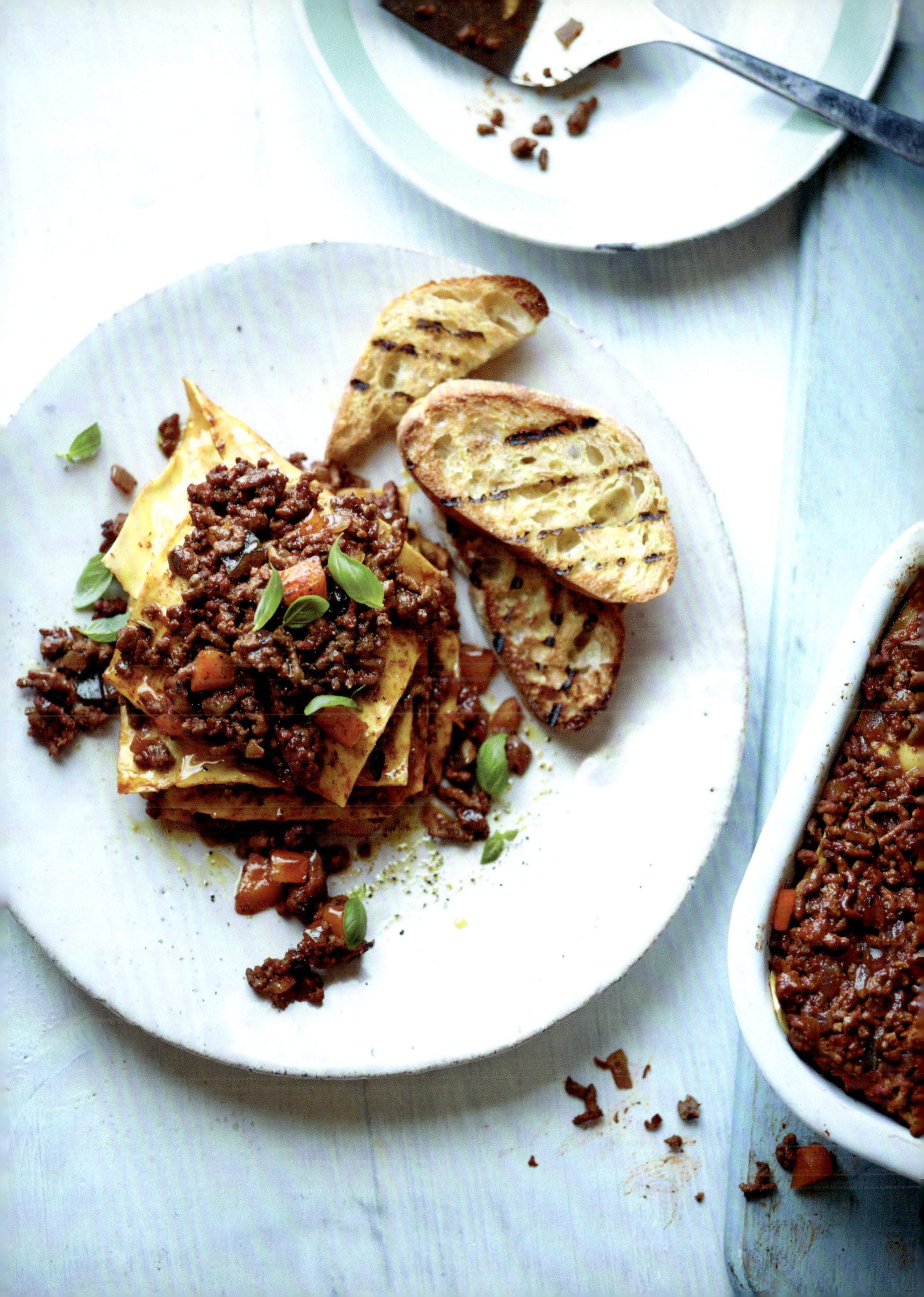

SERVES 2

SPANISH OMELETTE

This super-satisfying potato omelette needs about 30 minutes of your time, but it tastes great hot or cold, and so is perfect for carrying in a lunch box to work with some fresh salad.

LONGER RECIPE
MAKE AHEAD

INGREDIENTS

- 12 new potatoes
- 1 tbsp olive oil
- 5 spring onions, sliced
- 1 red chilli, thinly sliced – remove the seeds if you don't like it hot
- 2 handfuls of baby spinach leaves, plus a little extra to serve
- 300g deli-style cooked chicken or ham, roughly torn or sliced
- 8 eggs
- salt and pepper
- bread, to serve
- cherry tomatoes, to serve

METHOD

Prick the potatoes with a fork and microwave at 900w for 3 minutes. Leave them to rest for 2 minutes, then blast them for a further 2 minutes, by which time they should be cooked through. Leave to cool and then slice them up.

Preheat your grill to maximum.

Heat the olive oil in a decent non-stick frying pan (about 20cm in diameter) over a medium to high heat. Add the potatoes, and fry, turning every now and then, for 2 minutes. Add the spring onions and chilli and cook for another minute. Throw in the spinach, along with the chicken or ham, and fry for about 30 seconds or until the spinach has wilted.

Beat the eggs with a good pinch of salt and pepper, then pour into the frying pan. Use a wooden spoon or spatula to move the egg around, scraping it up from the base, for 1–2 minutes or until there is a good proportion of cooked egg in the pan. Leave the egg to cook for a minute longer, then slide the pan under the grill (if your frying pan has a plastic handle, make sure that this doesn't go under the grill!) and cook until the top of the omelette is just set.

Slide your omelette from the pan and cut it in half, then serve with a good chunk of bread and a side salad of the cherry tomatoes and the extra spinach.

SERVES 4

LONGER RECIPE
GOOD TO FREEZE

JOE'S SWEET POTATO COTTAGE PIE

Trust me, this dish takes a little while to cook (about 1 hour and 15 minutes), but the prep is easy and once you bang it in the oven, all you need is patience! The sweet potato topping makes this a real winner.

INGREDIENTS

- 4 sweet potatoes, peeled and cut into chunks
- salt and pepper
- 1 tbsp coconut oil
- 1kg reduced-fat (about 5%) beef mince
- 1 onion, roughly diced
- 1 red pepper, de-seeded and diced
- 2 carrots, grated
- 1 courgette, grated
- 2 tbsp tomato puree
- 200ml beef stock
- 75g frozen peas
- 3 tbsp Worcestershire sauce

METHOD

Preheat your oven to 200°C (fan 180°C, gas mark 6).

Bring a large saucepan of water to the boil. Add the sweet potato and simmer for about 10 minutes or until very tender. Drain in a colander, give them a little waft to get rid of some of the moisture, then tip back into the pan. Season generously with salt and pepper, then mash until reasonably smooth.

While the sweet potatoes are cooking, heat half of the coconut oil in a large frying pan or heavy-based casserole over a high heat. Add the mince and fry, breaking up any chunks, until the meat is just cooked and browned in places. Depending on the size of your pan, you may need to do this in two batches. Transfer the cooked meat to a bowl.

Heat the rest of the coconut oil in the same pan over a medium to high heat. Add the onion, red pepper, carrots and courgette and stir-fry for 5–6 minutes or until they just begin to soften. Squeeze in the tomato puree and cook, stirring, for a further 30 seconds, then tip the meat back in and stir well. Pour in the stock, bring to the boil and simmer for 20 minutes.

Remove from the heat and stir in the peas and Worcestershire sauce, then spoon into a large baking dish and top with the mashed sweet potato.

Bake your cottage pie for about 20 minutes, by which time the sweet potato topping should have crisped a little.

SPINACH AND TURKEY CANNELLONI

SERVES 4

LONGER RECIPE
MAKE AHEAD
GOOD TO FREEZE

INGREDIENTS

- 1½ tbsp olive oil
- 1 large red onion, diced
- 3 cloves garlic, finely chopped
- 1kg turkey mince
- 3 large handfuls of baby spinach leaves
- 300g ricotta
- salt and pepper
- 1 bunch of basil, leaves only, roughly chopped
- 16 dried cannelloni tubes
- 2 x 400g tins of chopped tomatoes
- crusty bread and a side salad, to serve

This is another batch-cooking winner. Invest an hour and 15 minutes of your time, then divide your cannelloni into 4 portions and you're all set for a few days. If you don't enjoy turkey mince, just use beef mince instead.

METHOD

Preheat your oven to 180°C (fan 160°C, gas mark 4).

Heat 1 tablespoon of the olive oil in a large frying pan over a medium to high heat. Add the onion and garlic and fry for 2 minutes, stirring regularly, until the onions are soft and taking on a little colour.

Increase the heat to high, add half of the turkey mince and fry for 2–3 minutes, breaking up any lumps with your spoon as you go. Cook the mince until there is no more pink left, then tip out into a bowl. Repeat the process with the remaining olive oil and turkey mince. When this second batch of mince is browned, toss the spinach into the pan and stir until wilted, then tip the whole lot into the bowl with the rest of the mince.

Add the ricotta to the bowl, along with a generous amount of salt and pepper and half of the basil, and mix everything together well. Using your fingers and a teaspoon, stuff the cannelloni tubes with the turkey mixture – don't worry about being perfect here, any overspill can just be added into the sauce later.

When all of the tubes are full, pour one of the tins of tomatoes into the base of a large baking dish (about 30cm x 18cm) and stir through any leftover turkey mixture. Now line up the stuffed cannelloni tubes in the dish and pour over the second tin of tomatoes, then cover the dish with foil.

Bake your cannelloni for 35–40 minutes, by which time the pasta should be cooked through. Remove from the oven, scatter with the rest of the basil and serve with a side salad and chunks of bread.

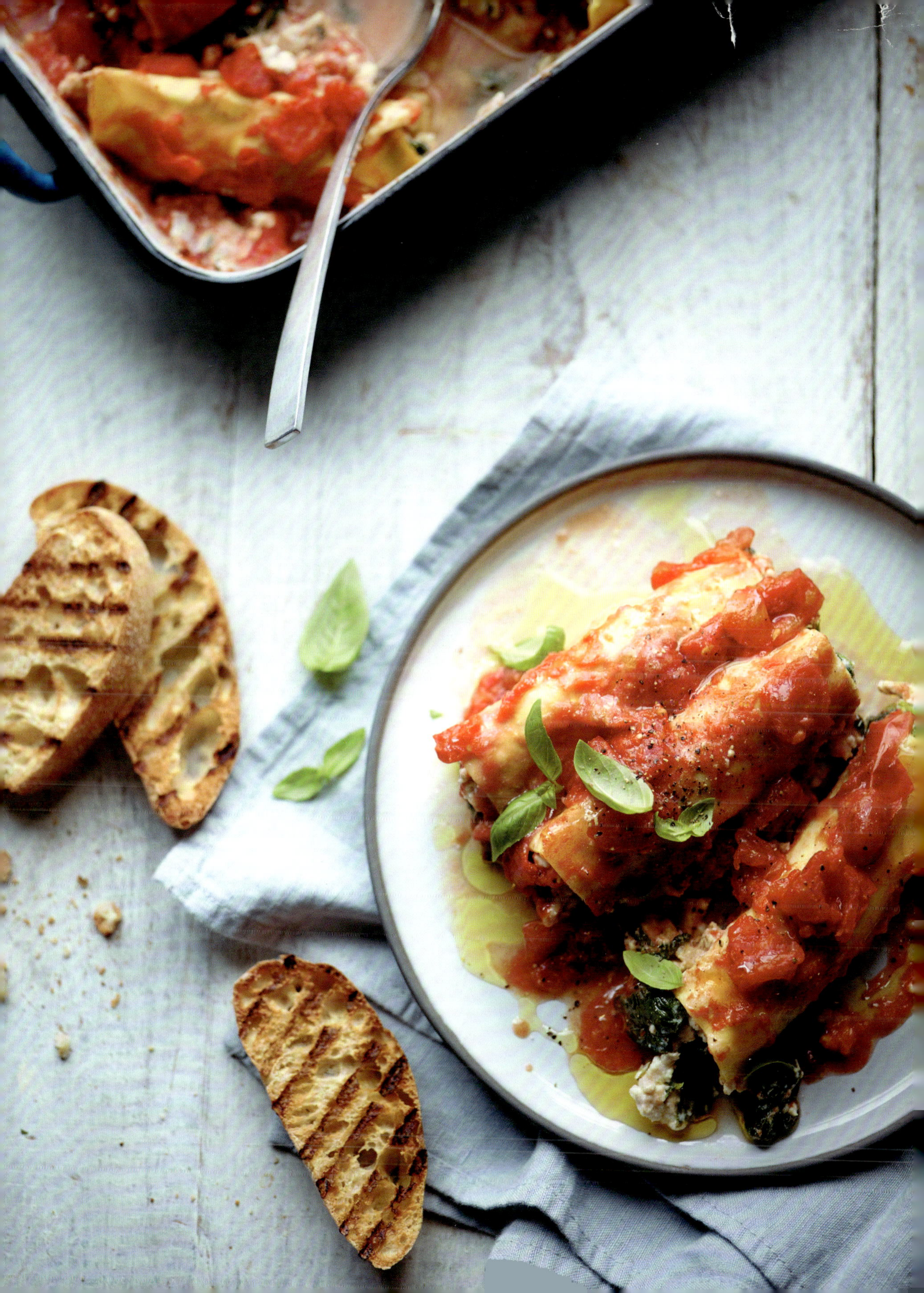

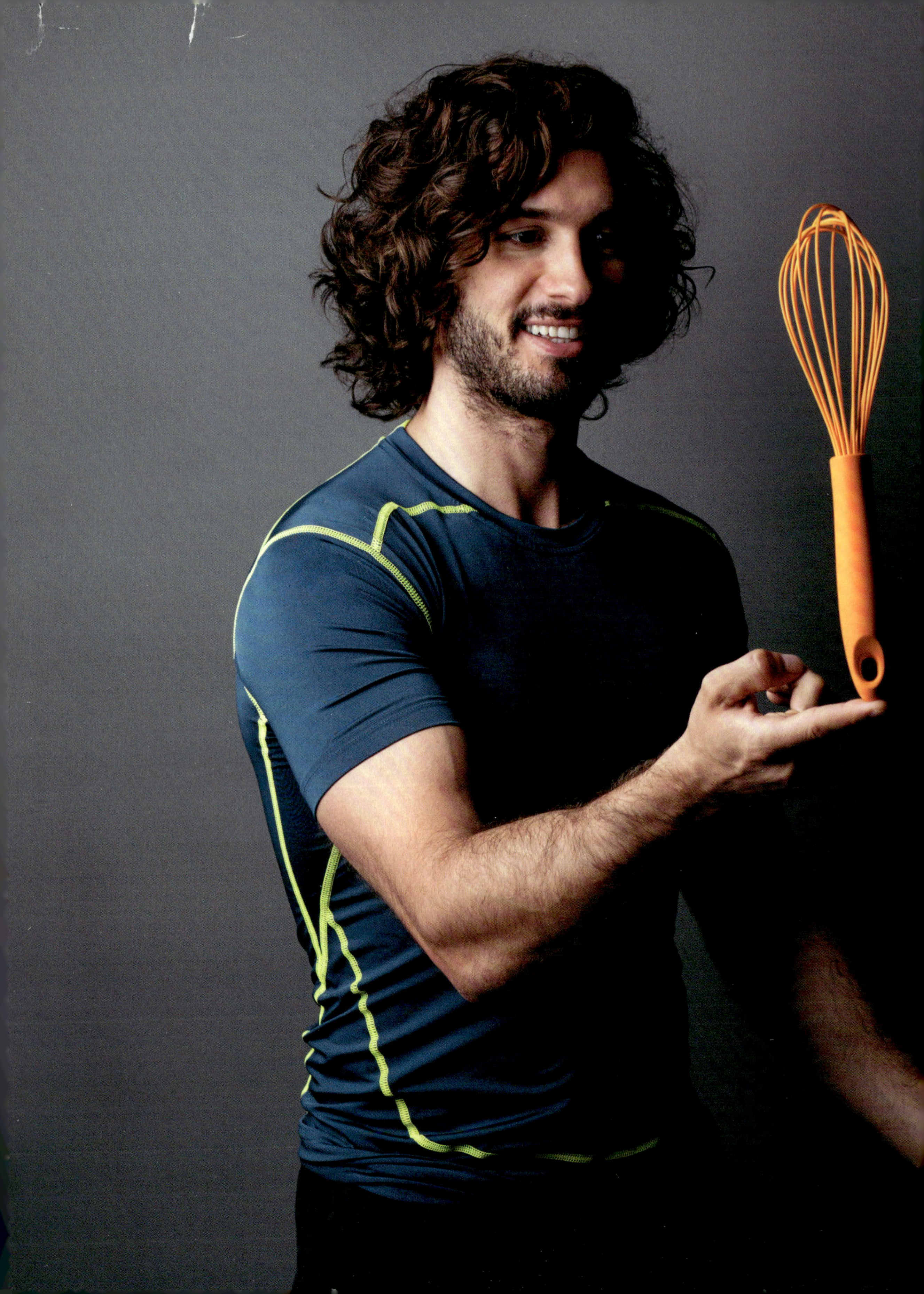

5

SNACKS AND TREATS

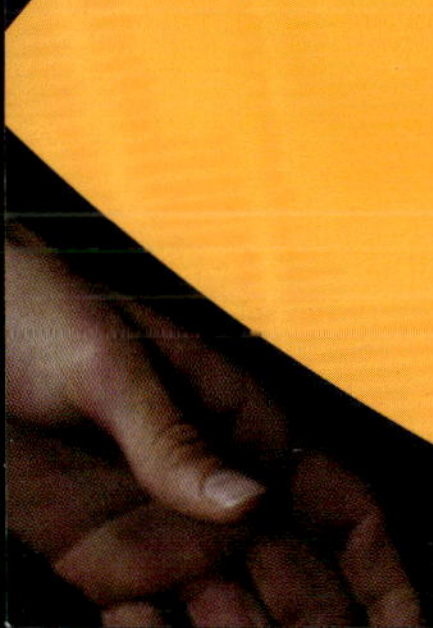

TUNA TARTARE

SERVES 2

If you like sushi, you will love this tartare. Good-quality fresh tuna should be fine to eat raw, but ask at your fishmonger or the fish counter in your local supermarket to be sure, letting them know you'll be eating the fish raw. Definitely give this dish a miss if you are pregnant or have a weakened immune system.

INGREDIENTS

- 4 tbsp rice wine vinegar
- 1 tsp salt
- ½ cucumber, de-seeded and cut into 1cm dice
- 400g raw tuna, cut into 1cm dice – or smaller if you can
- wholegrain rice cakes or rice crackers, to serve

METHOD

Pour the vinegar into a small bowl and thoroughly mix in the salt. Add the cucumber and leave to pickle for 5 minutes.

Drain off the vinegar and mix the lightly pickled cucumber with the tuna.

Serve up your raw fish treat with rice cakes or crackers for a delicious and different snack.

★ TOP TIP

You're working hard and training hard so why not treat yourself to one of my Lean in 15 treats? They're quite addictive, so don't get too greedy – share them with your friends! People are going to love you if you turn up to a party with healthy treats!

MAKES 2 LARGE FRITTERS

SWEETCORN AND FETA FRITTERS

These taste incredible and are very easy to make. They are good hot or cold, so you can make them the night before, ready to take to work in the morning. You can also double up the recipe and freeze half for another time.

MAKE AHEAD
GOOD TO FREEZE

INGREDIENTS

- 1 x 340g tin of sweetcorn, drained
- 1 red chilli, de-seeded and sliced, plus extra to serve – optional
- 3 spring onions, finely sliced
- 75g feta, crumbled
- 75g self-raising flour
- 1 egg
- salt and pepper
- 1 tbsp coconut oil
- 1 avocado, sliced
- juice of 1 lime, to serve
- drizzle of sesame oil – optional

METHOD

Place the sweetcorn, chilli (if using), spring onion, feta, flour, egg and 50ml of water in a large bowl. Season with salt and pepper, then mix until you have a lumpy batter.

Heat half of the coconut oil in a non-stick frying pan over a low to medium heat. When the oil is hot, spoon in half of the batter, spreading it evenly around the pan. Cook the batter for about 2 minutes without flipping or budging . . . that's about time for 20 press-ups!

Flip the fritter and cook for a further 2 minutes. Remove from the pan and transfer to paper towels to drain off any excess oil while you cook the second fritter.

Serve the fritters with the avocado, a good squeeze of lime juice and, if you like, a drizzle of sesame oil and a sprinkling of chilli (see picture overleaf).

TUNA AND COURGETTE FRITTERS

MAKES 12–14 SMALL (or 4 big)

MAKE AHEAD
GOOD TO FREEZE

INGREDIENTS

1 x 160g tin of tuna, drained
1 courgette, grated
80g self-raising flour
1 egg
1 tbsp coconut oil
light soy sauce, to serve

Such an awesome and tasty snack – and there's nearly always a spare tin of tuna knocking about in the cupboard. You can batch-cook and freeze these too, if you like.

METHOD

Flake the tuna out of the tin into a bowl, then add the courgette, flour and egg. Mix together to make a batter. If need be, add a dribble of water to loosen the consistency until it resembles thick double cream.

Melt a little of the oil in a frying pan over a medium heat. Spoon in large mounds of the batter, leaving some space between each one, as the batter will spread and work itself into a little puddle. Aim for fritters about 7–8cm in diameter if you want to make about a dozen – but feel free to just make four big ones instead.

Cook the fritters for about 2–3 minutes on each side before lifting them out of the pan and draining on paper towels.

Serve the fritters with a small bowl of soy sauce for dipping.

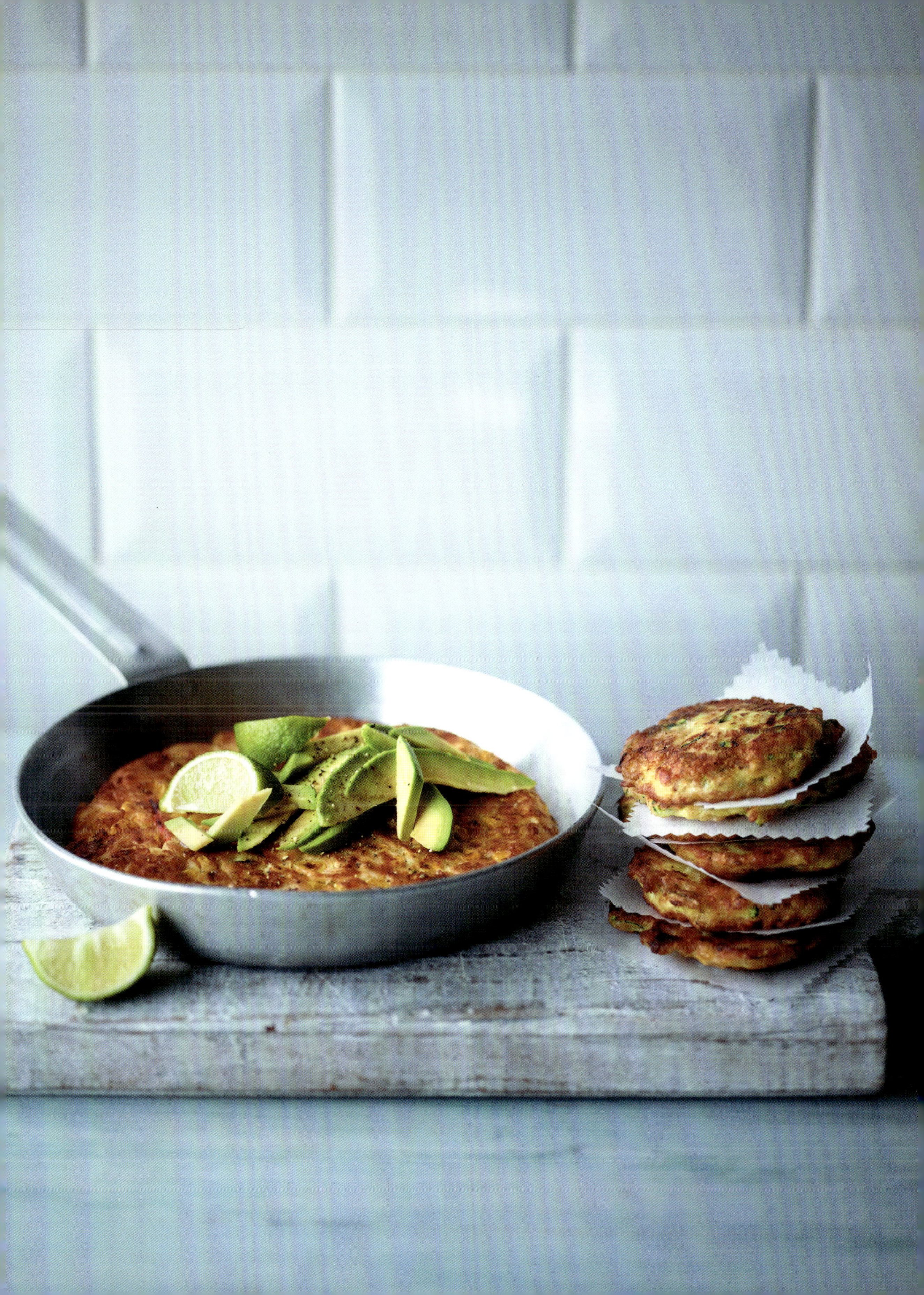

MAKES 400g

INGREDIENTS

400g cashew nuts
2 tsp olive or groundnut oil
2 tsp ground cumin
1½ tsp smoked paprika

SPICED CASHEWS

METHOD

Preheat your oven to 190°C (fan 170°C, gas mark 5).

Mix all the ingredients together, then tip onto a baking tray and roast in the oven for 12–15 minutes until the nuts are crisp and lightly coloured. Remove from the oven and sprinkle with salt. These spiced nuts will keep in an airtight container for up to 5 days.

MAKES 400g

INGREDIENTS

400g unsalted peanuts
4 tsp wasabi powder
2 tsp olive oil

WASABI PEANUTS

METHOD

Preheat your oven to 190°C (fan 170°C, gas mark 5).

Mix all the ingredients together, then tip onto a baking tray and roast in the oven for 12–15 minutes until the nuts are crisp and lightly coloured. Remove from the oven and sprinkle with salt. The wasabi nuts will keep in an airtight container for up to 4 days.

MAKES 24

INGREDIENTS

3 mini tortilla wraps
a few pumps of olive oil spray
2 tsp ground cumin
1 tsp smoked paprika
1 tsp celery salt

SPICED TORTILLA CHIPS

METHOD

Preheat your oven to 170°C (fan 150°C, gas mark 3).

Take each tortilla in turn and give it a pump of oil on both sides. Cut the tortilla into quarters, then cut each quarter in half to give you 8 triangles. Lay as many of the 24 triangles onto a baking tray as you can fit (you might have to use a couple of trays, or cook the tortilla chips in two batches).

Mix together the spices and salt until they are all well blended, then sprinkle evenly over the triangles. Bake in the oven for 6–7 minutes until lightly golden and crisp.

★ **TOP TIP**

Nuts are great for a party – and much healthier for you than something like crisps! But they're still a treat, so don't get too carried away. I recommend a portion of 20–30g, no more than once a day.

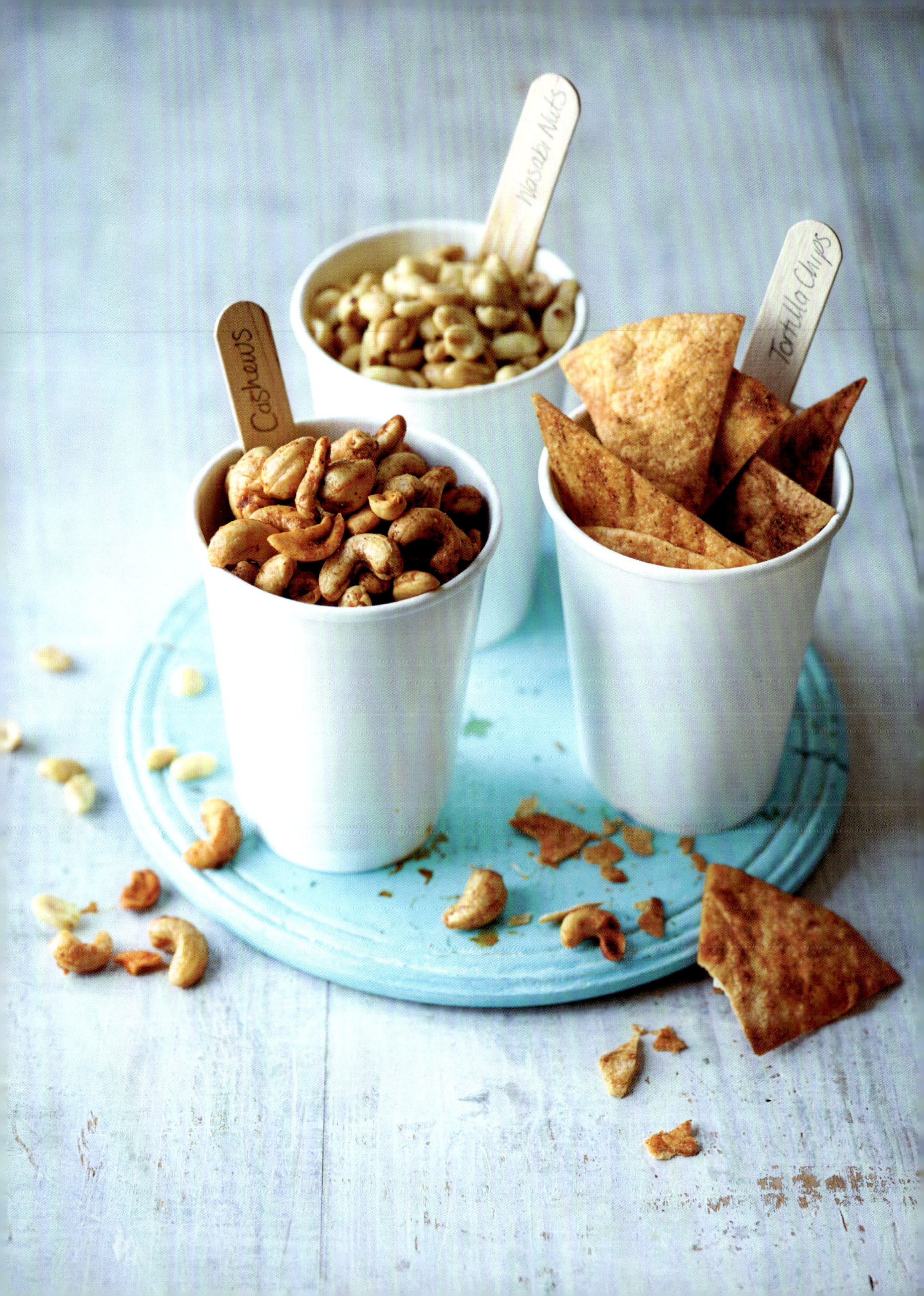
Wasabi Nuts
Tortilla Chips
Cashews

SERVES 2

MAKE AHEAD

INGREDIENTS

- 2 heads of broccoli, broken into florets
- 4 tbsp pine nuts
- 3 tbsp finely grated parmesan
- 2 bunches of basil, leaves only
- 1 clove garlic, roughly chopped
- juice and finely grated zest of 1 lemon
- 75ml olive oil
- salt and pepper
- chopped raw vegetables, to serve

MIDGET TREE AND PINE NUT PESTO

This is a great snack that will keep in an airtight container in the fridge for up to 3 days. Other green veg, such as kale and spinach, work well too. I like to eat this with chopped cauliflower, carrot and cucumber for dipping.

METHOD

Bring a saucepan of water to the boil. Drop in the broccoli florets and cook for 1 minute. Drain in a sieve or colander, then rinse under cold running water.

Tip the broccoli into a blender and add the pine nuts, parmesan, basil, garlic, lemon juice and zest and olive oil. Season generously with salt and pepper, then pulse until virtually smooth – you will most likely have to do quite a bit of pulsing and scraping.

Serve the pesto with chopped raw vegetables.

SERVES 2

INGREDIENTS

- 180g cream cheese
- 2 tbsp chopped chives
- 2 tbsp chopped tarragon
- 2 tbsp chopped basil
- 1 small clove garlic, finely sliced
- 6 sundried tomatoes, roughly chopped
- 50g walnuts, roughly crumbled
- celery, carrot and cucumber sticks, to serve

WHIPPED-UP HERBY CREAM CHEESE

This is the perfect cheese-lover's snack, and the fresh herbs used in combination are a real winner. This can be made by hand if you don't have a food processor – it just takes a bit more time.

METHOD

Place all the ingredients except the walnuts and the vegetable sticks in a food processor, along with about 2 tablespoons of warm water. Blitz until totally smooth.

Tip the dip into a bowl, top with the walnuts and then dig in with the celery, carrot and cucumber 'spades'.

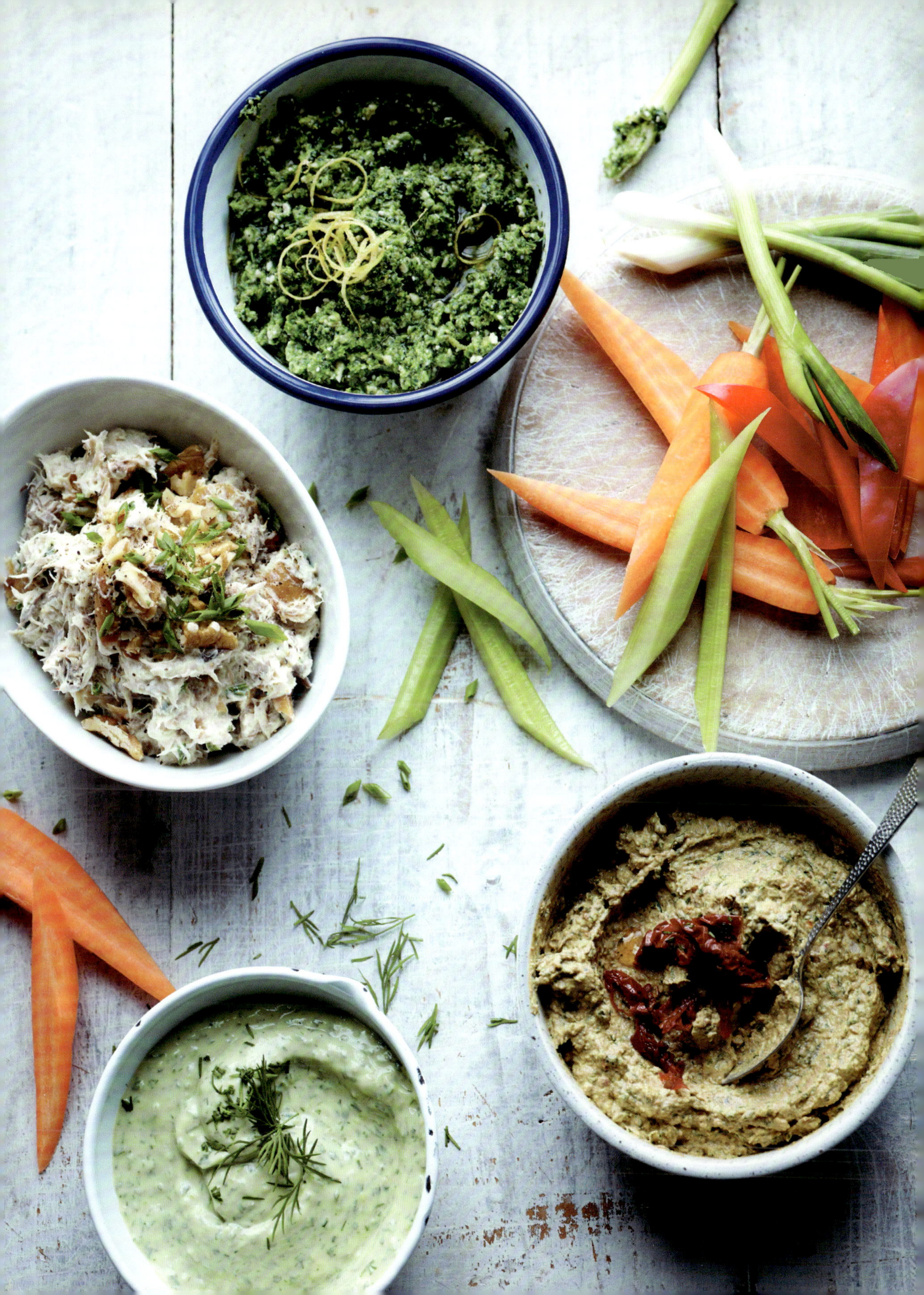

SMOKED MACKEREL PÂTÉ

SERVES 4

Raw cauliflower florets taste amazing with this pâté, which can be kept in an airtight container in the fridge for up to 4 days.

INGREDIENTS

300g smoked mackerel
75g crème fraiche
juice of 1 lemon
freshly ground black pepper
small bunch of chives, finely sliced
35g walnuts, roughly chopped
chopped carrots, cauliflower florets and sliced red pepper, to serve

METHOD

Remove the skin from the mackerel and, using your fingers, flake the fish into small pieces. Add the crème fraiche and lemon juice, along with a good grinding of black pepper. Use a fork to mix and mash until you're happy with the consistency of your pâté – I like it with a bit of texture.

Stir in the chives, then top the pâté with the walnuts. Serve with the carrots, cauliflower and red pepper.

AVOCADO RANCH WITH DIPPING STICKS

SERVES 2

If you love avocado, this creamy ranch dip will be right up your street. It only takes about 5 minutes to make and is jam-packed with healthy fats to keep you energized.

INGREDIENTS

1 large avocado, roughly chopped
245g full-fat Greek yoghurt
juice of 1 lemon
1 clove garlic, grated or finely chopped
small handful of chives, finely chopped
small handful of dill, finely chopped
small handful of parsley, finely chopped
salt and pepper
6 large celery sticks, to serve

METHOD

Place the avocado in a food processor. Add the yoghurt, lemon juice, garlic, chives, dill and parsley. Season with salt and pepper, then process until smooth.

Serve the avocado dip with the celery sticks.

★ **TOP TIP**

SNACK IDEAS

If you don't have time to make a snack, here are a few ideas for you!

- ★ Scoop of whey protein with water
- ★ 20–30g nuts
- ★ 85g beef jerky
- ★ Boiled egg
- ★ 75–100g fruit (melon, blueberries, strawberries, raspberries, apple or pear). Please limit fruit to one snack per day and try not to have it more than a few times a week because it won't help your fat-burning.

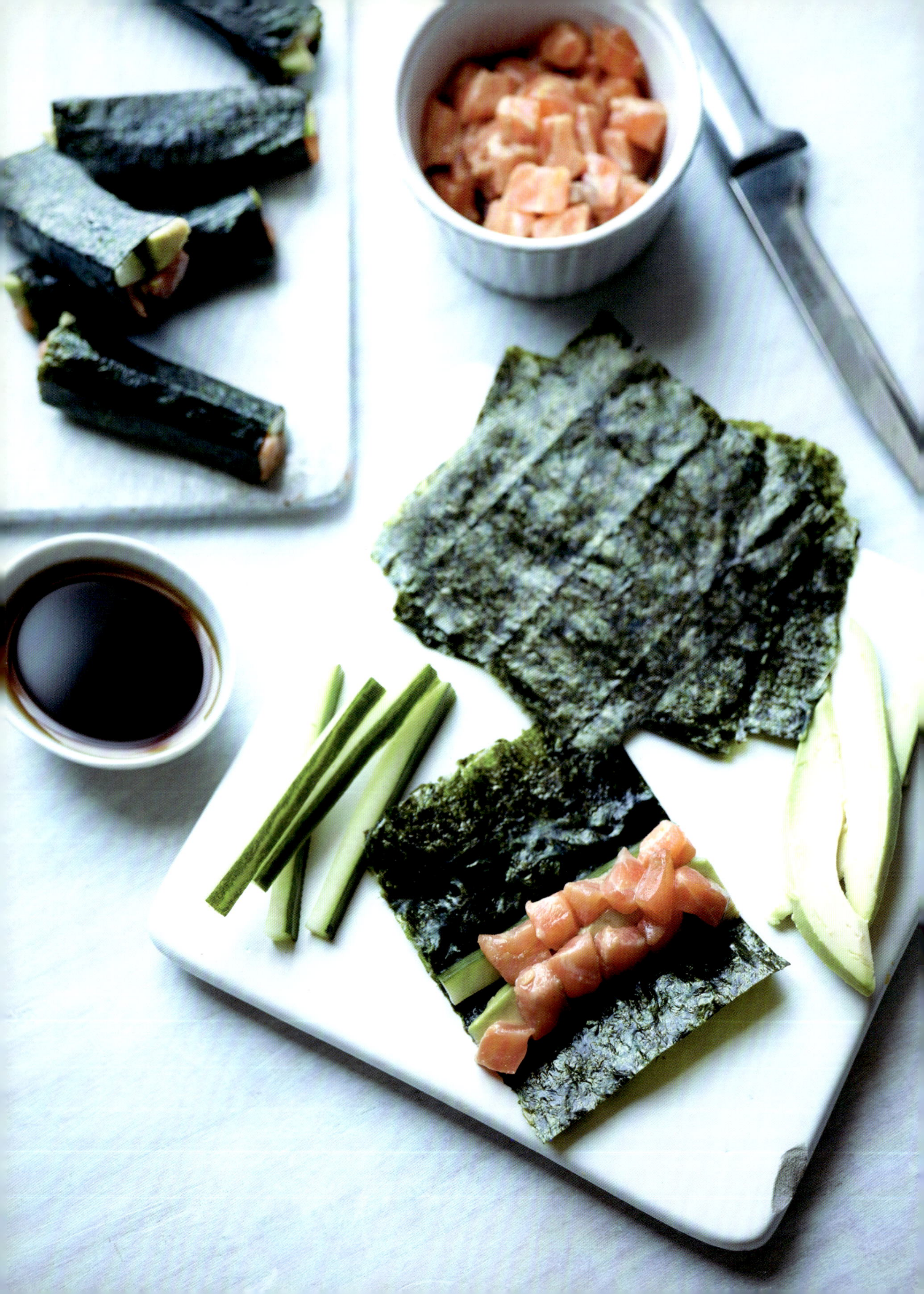

SALMON AND AVOCADO HAND ROLL

Another great snack option that's high in healthy fats. This dish is so impressive you could easily serve it as a starter at a dinner party. Just make sure you get the very freshest fish from your fishmonger – let them know you'll be serving it raw. Anyone with a compromised immune system should avoid raw fish altogether, as should pregnant women.

SERVES 2

INGREDIENTS

- 400g raw salmon, cut into 1cm dice – or smaller if possible
- 1cm ginger, finely grated
- 1½ tbsp light soy sauce
- 2 tsp sesame oil
- 2 tsp rice wine vinegar
- 1 avocado, halved and peeled
- 2 large sheets of nori seaweed (about 20cm x 20cm)
- ¼ cucumber, de-seeded and sliced into 8 batons

METHOD

Place the salmon, ginger, soy sauce, sesame oil and vinegar in a bowl and mix well.

Cut each avocado half lengthways into 4 slices, so you have 8 slices of avocado.

Cut each sheet of nori into 4 equal squares.

Spread out your nori squares and lay a slice of avocado in the middle of each one, then sit a cucumber baton alongside. Divide the salmon mixture evenly among the squares of nori, spooning it along the length of the avocado and cucumber.

Dip a finger in some water and dampen the edge of the nori squares so that they will stick.

Roll up your hand rolls and prepare to enjoy a Zen-like taste experience.

BEETROOT PROTEIN BROWNIES

MAKES ABOUT 16

LONGER RECIPE

INGREDIENTS

2 cooked and peeled beetroot (about 140g), roughly chopped
175g ground almonds
120g chestnut puree
30g cocoa powder
45g honey
1 scoop (30g) vanilla protein powder
2 tsp vanilla extract
4 eggs

I didn't want to release a cookbook without a few sweet treats. These are yummy, and way healthier than your normal chocolate brownies. But they should still be enjoyed on occasion and not scoffed every day. A slice once a week, after a workout, is fine. These take more like 30 minutes than 15 minutes to make – but hey, you have to earn your treats!

METHOD

Preheat your oven to 180°C (fan 160°C, gas mark 4).

Place all the ingredients in a food processor and blitz to a smooth batter.

Tip the batter into a lined brownie tin (about 28cm x 15cm) and bake for 18 minutes.

Remove the brownie from the oven and leave to cool slightly before cutting into squares and chomping down.

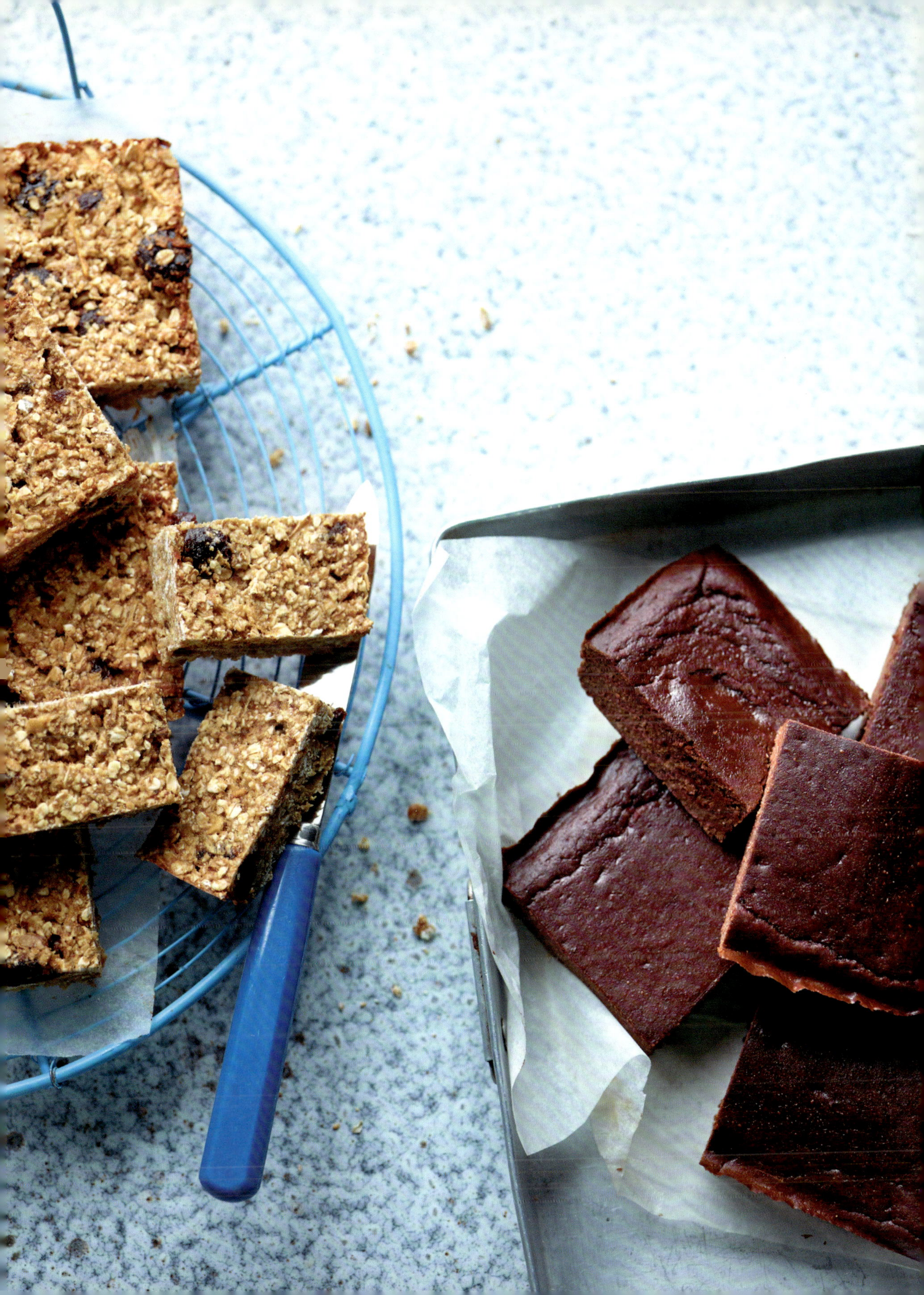

POST-WORKOUT POWER SQUARES

MAKES 24 SQUARES

LONGER RECIPE
MAKE AHEAD

INGREDIENTS

12 pitted dates
100g rice cakes
220g rolled oats
1 scoop (30g) vanilla protein powder
2 apples, cored and grated
½ tsp baking powder
100g dried cherries, halved

Here's another tasty treat that can be whipped up inside half an hour. But don't forget these aren't for everyday eating. Enjoy them no more than once a week and share them with friends, so you don't scoff all 24 on your own! There's no excuse for 'eating them up' so they won't go to waste either, as they'll last for 5 days in an airtight container.

METHOD

Preheat your oven to 160°C (fan 140°C, gas mark 3).

Bring the kettle to the boil. Cover the dates with boiling water and leave to soak for 5 minutes.

Blitz the rice cakes in a food processor until they are totally broken down into fine crumbs. Tip them out into a large bowl.

Drain the dates, blitz in the food processor until smooth and add to the bowl with the rice cakes, along with the remaining ingredients. Mix everything together until thoroughly combined – the mixture can be a bit stiff, so get your hands in there if need be.

Tip the mixture into a lined brownie tin (about 28cm x 15cm) and bake for 25 minutes. Leave to cool before cutting into squares.

JOE'S GRANOLA

MAKES A DECENT JARFUL

LONGER RECIPE
MAKE AHEAD

INGREDIENTS

- 175g mixed nuts – I like cashews, pecans, walnuts, almonds
- 1 tsp ground cinnamon
- 1 apple, cored and grated, skin and all
- 150g rolled oats
- 20g honey
- 40g raisins

Why buy sugary processed granolas when, with half an hour to spare, you can make your own healthy version at home? This goes really well with Greek yoghurt and some fresh berries at breakfast time. Don't rely on it every day, though. Nothing beats eggs for breakfast.

METHOD

Preheat your oven to 180°C (fan 160°C, gas mark 4).

Mix all the ingredients except the raisins in a large bowl, then tip onto a large baking tray, spreading it out into a single layer.

Bake for 25 minutes, pulling out the tray a couple of times and mixing everything around so the granola toasts evenly.

Remove from the oven and leave to cool before stirring in the raisins. The granola will keep in a well-sealed jar for at least 2 days – although I bet it doesn't last that long!

SERVES
1

LONGER RECIPE

JOE'S PROTEIN RICE PUDDING

If you have a sweet tooth, then this is a nice snack to enjoy after a workout, particularly with some fresh berries. Allow about half an hour to make this one.

INGREDIENTS

100g pudding rice
500ml almond milk
1 tbsp honey
1 scoop (30g) vanilla protein powder

METHOD

Place the rice, almond milk, honey and 150ml of water in a saucepan. Bring to the boil and simmer for 20–25 minutes, stirring regularly, especially towards the end, when it will become creamy and thick.

Remove from the heat and leave to cool a little before stirring through the protein powder. Do not add the protein powder with the pan on the heat, or the whey will cook and go lumpy.

Eat the pudding straight away. Or, for a more indulgent finish, pour into a baking dish and place under a hot grill until the top is nicely browned and lightly crisp.

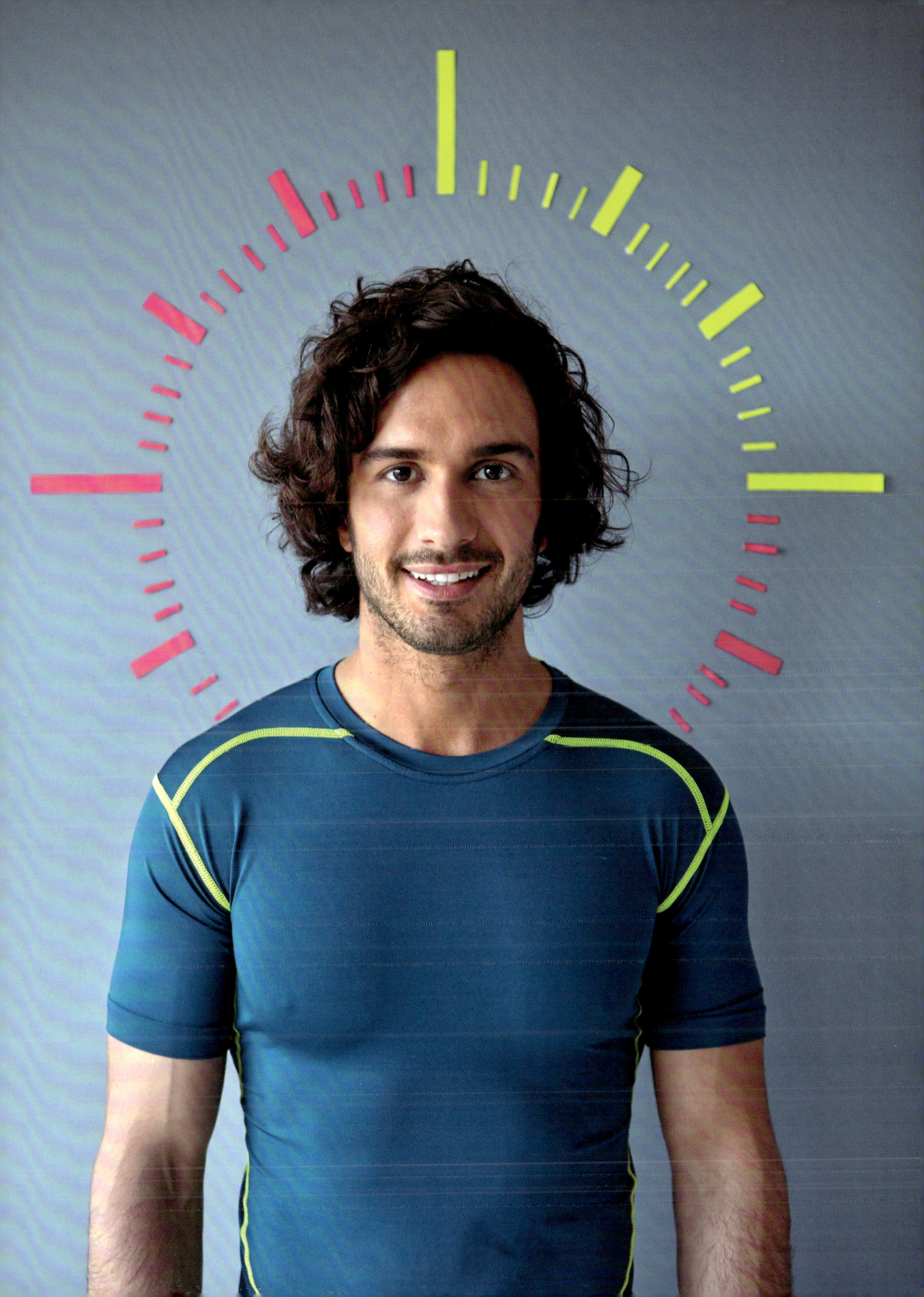

BANANA AND PECAN CUPCAKES

MAKES 12

LONGER RECIPE
MAKE AHEAD

INGREDIENTS

100g pecans, plus 12 extra for decorating
70g chestnut puree
3 very ripe bananas, peeled and roughly sliced (you need about 190g flesh)
30g honey
1 scoop (30g) vanilla protein powder
2 tsp vanilla extract
50g ground almonds
4 eggs
12 tsp crème fraiche

Ready in 20 minutes, these are my favourite treat and quite addictive, so again go easy on them. You won't burn fat eating them every day, so save them for a special treat or make them for a party with friends. The blacker the banana, the better – seriously, totally black is fine for these.

METHOD

Preheat the oven to 190°C (fan 170°C, gas mark 5) and line a 12-hole cupcake tin with paper cases.

Place all the ingredients except the extra pecans and the crème fraiche in a food processor and blend until you have a smooth, runny batter.

Divide the batter evenly between the cupcake cases and bake for 18 minutes, or until risen and lightly golden on top.

Leave to cool, then decorate each cupcake with a teaspoon of crème fraiche and a pecan.

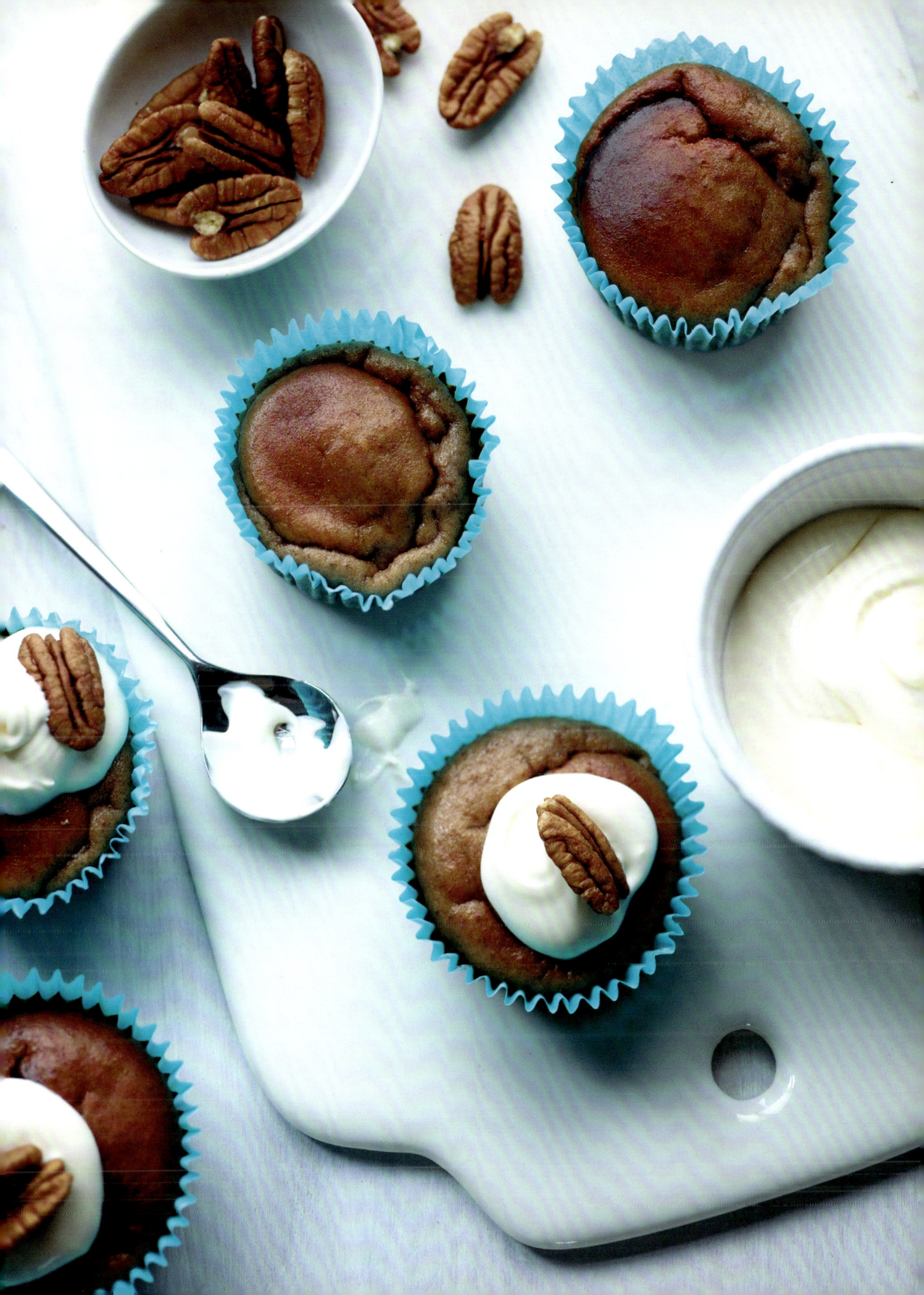

CHEAT'S BANANA AND ALMOND ICE CREAM

SERVES 2

LONGER RECIPE
(quick to make, but needs 4 hours in the freezer)
MAKE AHEAD

I love ice cream, so I thought I would share this healthier cheat's ice cream recipe with you. Feel free to add other frozen fruit, such as strawberries or raspberries, to mix up the flavour.

INGREDIENTS

- 4 bananas, peeled and cut into roughly similar-sized chunks
- 1 tbsp almond butter
- 50ml almond milk
- 1 scoop (30g) vanilla protein powder
- toasted flaked almonds, to serve – optional

METHOD

Line a baking tray with greaseproof paper and spread the banana chunks over it in a single layer. Place the tray in your freezer and freeze for a minimum of 4 hours, or until the banana chunks are frozen solid.

Tip the frozen banana into a food processor, along with the almond butter, almond milk and the protein powder, then pulse until virtually smooth.

Serve your cheat's ice cream topped with the toasted almonds, if using.

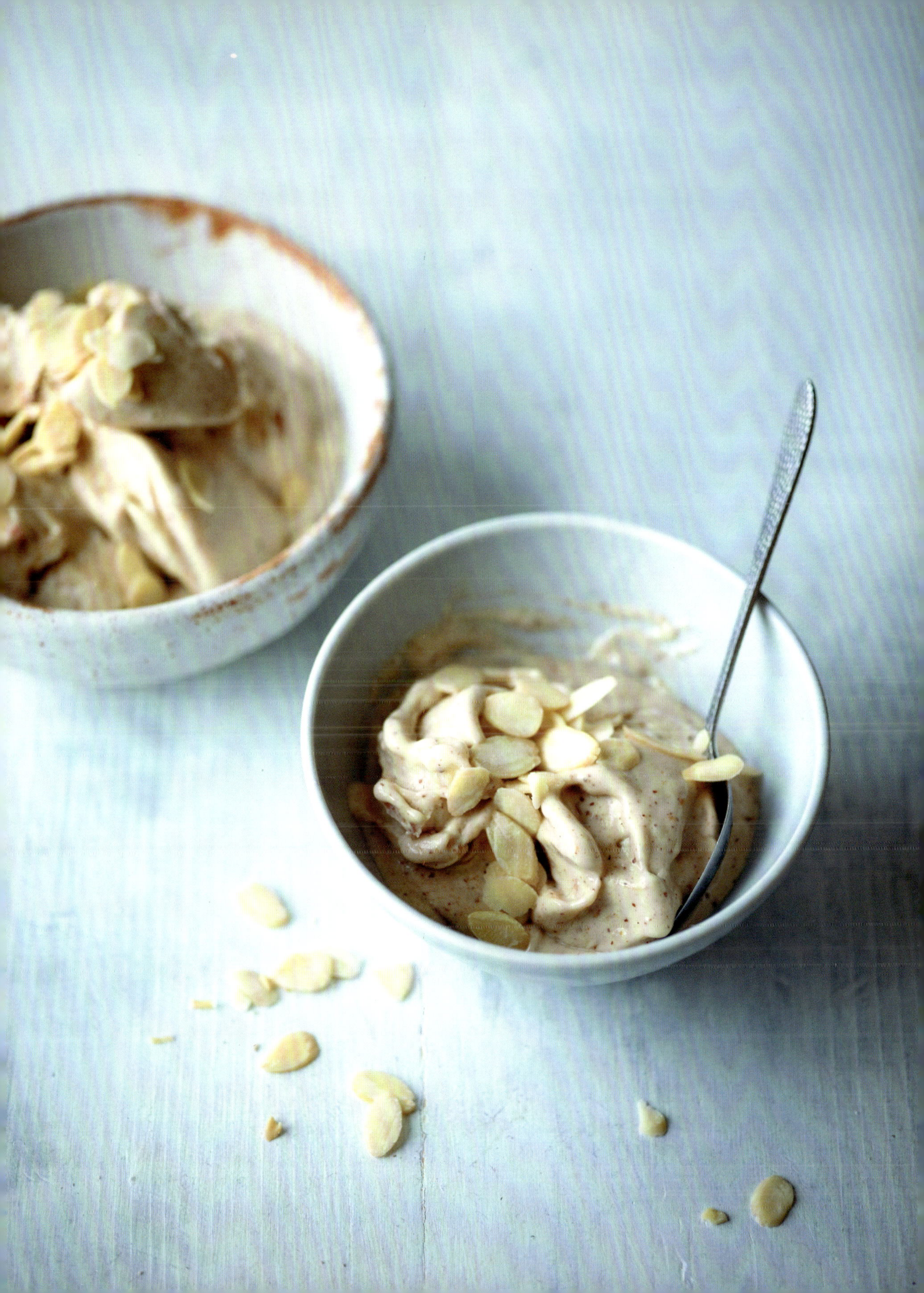

CHOCOLATE AND ALMOND PROTEIN CAKE

SERVES 6

LONGER RECIPE
MAKE AHEAD

INGREDIENTS

120g pitted dates
125g chestnut puree
10g cocoa powder, plus a little extra for dusting
100g ground almonds
100g chocolate (85% cocoa), melted
2 scoops (60g) vanilla protein powder
4 eggs
juice and finely grated zest of 1 orange

Well, I can't pretend this is particularly healthy, but everyone needs a treat sometimes – and, as treats go, this one is packed with nutritional goodness! The higher the percentage of cocoa in chocolate, the better it is for you – I've gone for 85% here. And if you don't have chestnut puree, feel free to substitute almond butter. You'll need to allow 30 minutes to make this cake.

METHOD

Preheat your oven to 180°C (fan 160°C, gas mark 4) and line a 23cm round cake tin with baking parchment.

Bring the kettle to the boil. Pour 150ml of boiling water over the dates and leave to soak for 5 minutes.

Tip the soaked dates, along with their soaking water, into a food processor and puree until smooth. Then add the remaining ingredients and blitz into a smooth batter.

Pour the batter into the prepared tin and bake for 20 minutes. The cake will rise in the oven, but collapse again as it cools.

Remove the cake from the tin, dust with the extra cocoa powder . . . and head to the gym for a workout, so you can properly enjoy your treat afterwards!

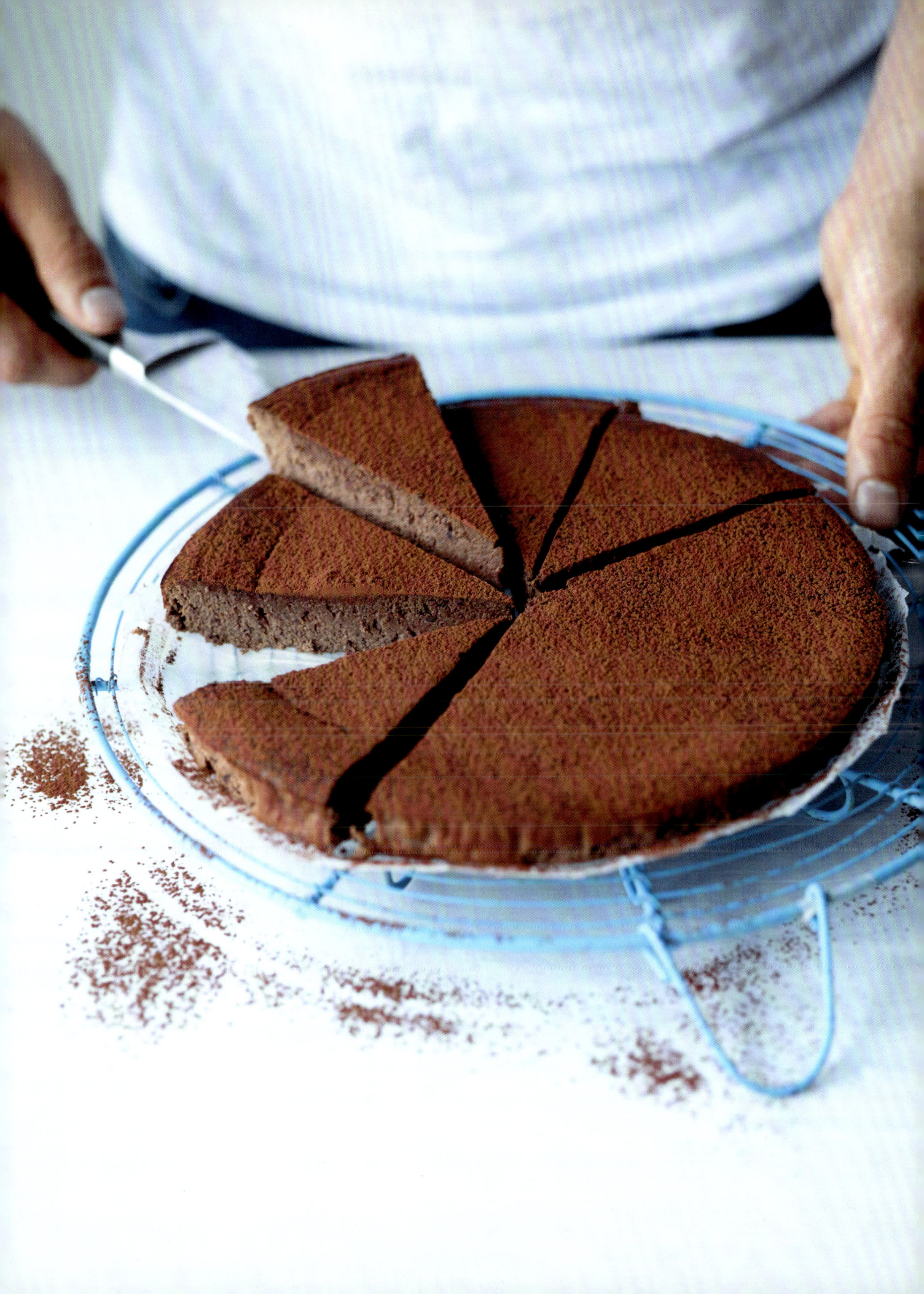

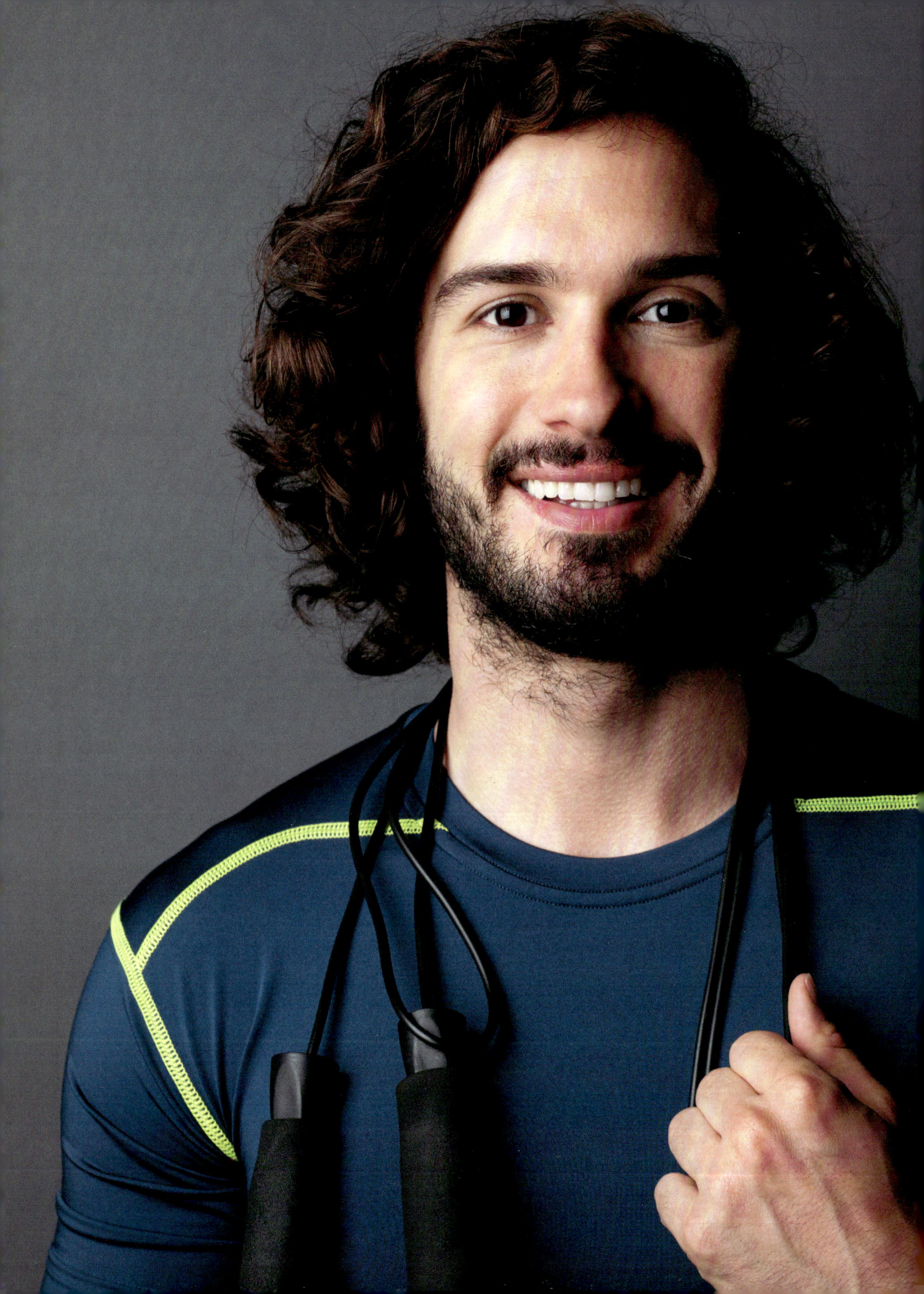

6

BURN FAT AND BUILD LEAN MUSCLE WITH HIIT

HIGH INTENSITY INTERVAL TRAINING (HIIT)

HIIT is one of the most effective training methods for burning fat. It might sound a bit scary, but it's not, as it's all relative to your own fitness and abilities. Everyone on my 90 Day Shift, Shape and Sustain plan, regardless of age or fitness levels, does it – with incredible results. Not only does it burn fat fast, but it also gets you outrageously fit by massively improving your cardiovascular fitness. Every session should be hard work, but the good news is it's all over in less than 20 minutes and you will feel like an absolute winner after each session. And when your body fat melts away, it's all worth it.

WHAT IS IT?

HIIT involves short bursts of maximal effort, followed by recovery periods of low-intensity activity or rest, i.e. 20 seconds of work, followed by 40 seconds of rest. You repeat this for 15–20 minutes and that's it. Job done. Bye bye, body fat!

As I said, it's all relative to your fitness levels, so let's take a treadmill, for example: if you're a beginner, HIIT could mean an incline power walk or a jog; if you're much fitter, then it could mean a sprint. The aim is to elevate your heart rate to near maximum during the intense working sets, before letting it recover in the rest periods.

> ‘Get in the zone, focus and train like a super-hero!’

Unlike low-intensity cardio, such as steady jogging, which only burns calories during the actual workout, HIIT burns calories for up to 18 hours afterwards. This is known as the after-burn effect, where your body is working hard to repay the oxygen debt in your system and restore itself to a resting state. During this time your metabolic rate is elevated, so your body burns more calories and therefore more fat. The more intense your workout, the greater your oxygen debt will be, so you should always aim to push yourself as hard as possible. Check with your doctor first if you have any health issues. If you can talk, text or tweet during a HIIT session, then you aren't working hard enough – so get in the zone, focus and train like a super-hero!

HOW DO I DO IT?

HIIT principles can be applied to any cardio machine, such as a treadmill, cross-trainer, rowing machine or exercise bike, or to body-weight exercises like burpees, mountain climbers, skipping or sprints.

Choose an exercise or combination of exercises that are suitable for you and which challenge you. You could do the same type of HIIT each time or you can change it up, i.e. rowing machine one day and then cross-trainer the next. As long as you are working hard and enjoying your training, it's all good.

WARM UP

Always carry out an exercise-specific warm up before starting your HIIT. For example, if you are going to do treadmill sprints, I recommend a power walk or slow jog before you start to sprint. The aim of a warm up is to prime your muscles and joints for the exercise they're about to perform. This is really important to prevent injuries and ensure you get the most out of your workouts, so don't be naughty and skip your warm up!

WORKOUT

Once you've warmed up, you can start your HIIT. I find the most effective protocol is a work:rest ratio of 1:2, meaning you rest for twice as long as you work. This allows you to really smash your working set and get a good recovery.

FOR EXAMPLE

Working set of 20 seconds
with a resting set of 40 seconds

OR

Working set of 30 seconds
with a resting set of 45 or 60 seconds

The effort must come in the working sets, so choose the timings that best suit you. During the resting sets, you can either slow down or come to a complete stop. You will repeat this for 15–20 minutes. It may not seem like much – but trust me, this is enough to create a calorie deficit. And if you fuel your body with the right macronutrients, you will start to see your body transform. Remember that over-training is NOT necessary, so don't get all carried away by doing two HIIT sessions per day. This will actually be counterproductive for your fat loss. Do one session, do it properly, and you won't want to do it again!

'DO ONE SESSION, DO IT PROPERLY, AND YOU WON'T WANT TO DO IT AGAIN!'

Here are two workouts for you to try out at home. My advice would be to do both workouts twice each week (so four in total), then add in an extra HIIT, if you fancy it.

WORKOUT 1: *CARDIO HIIT*

This workout involves three body-weight exercises that are guaranteed to get your heart rate up and your body fat melting. You need no equipment and only a small space, so you could do this in the garden or living room.

1. **High knees**
2. **Mountain climbers**
3. **Burpees**

1. **20 seconds High knees**
 40 seconds rest

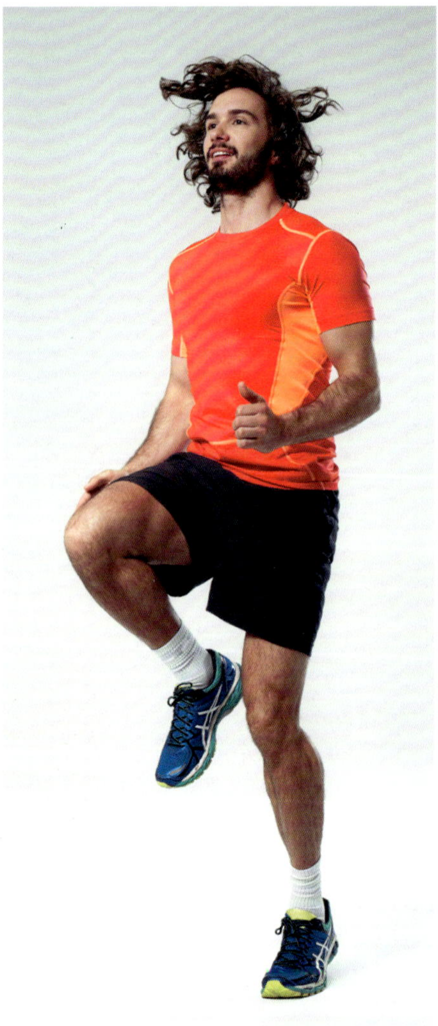

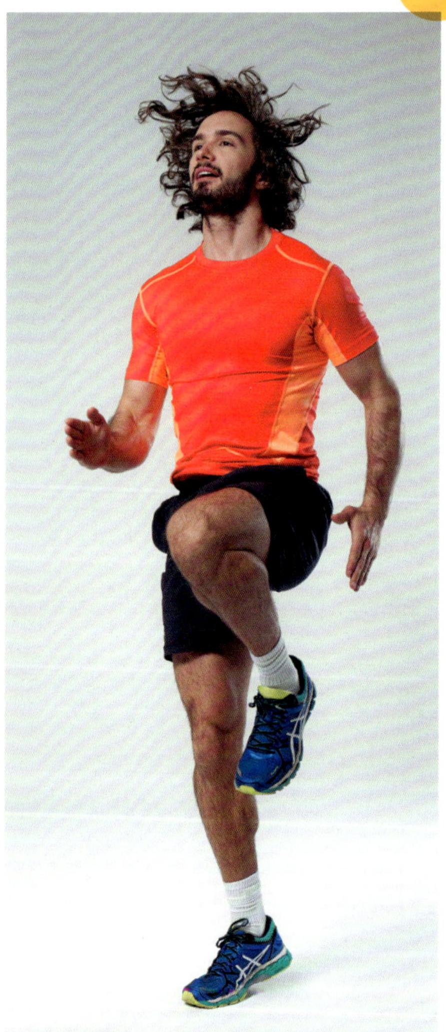

2. 20 seconds Mountain climbers

40 seconds rest

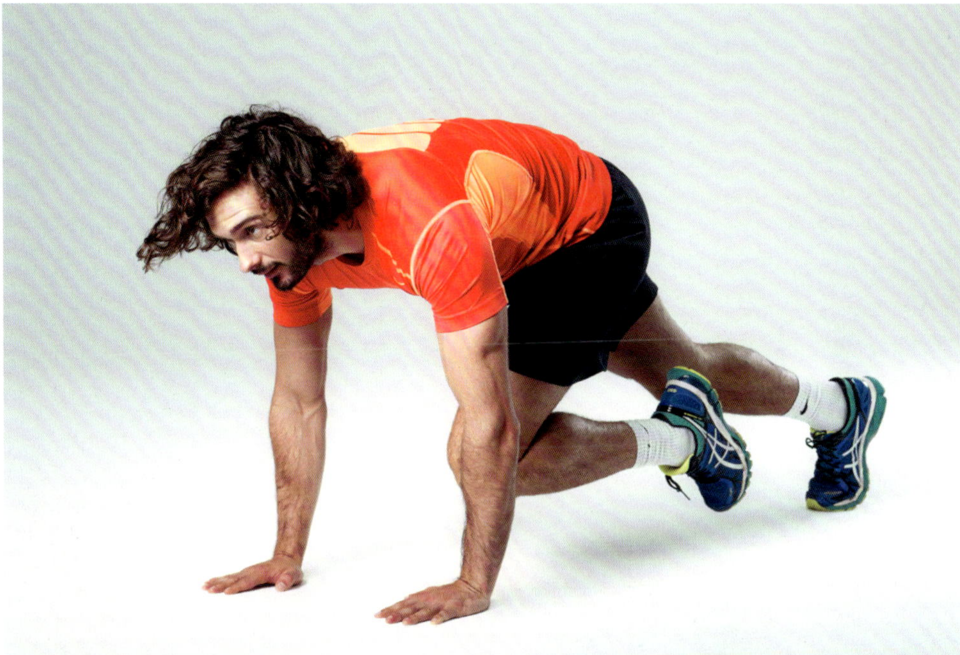

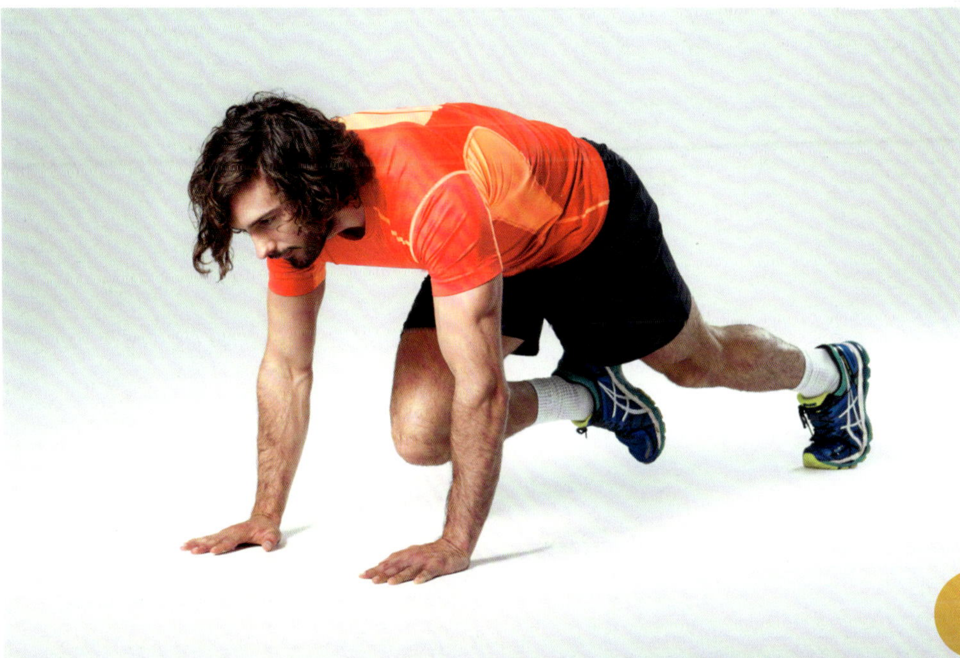

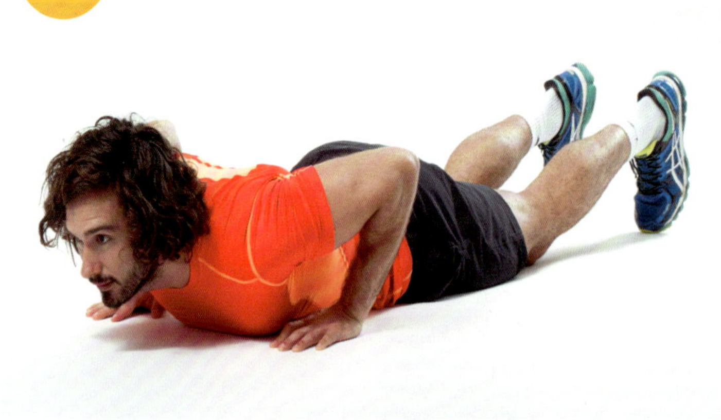

3. **20 seconds Burpees**

40 seconds rest

Repeat this circuit 5 times, making a total of 15 minutes. If you find this too easy, work for 30 seconds and rest for 30 seconds.

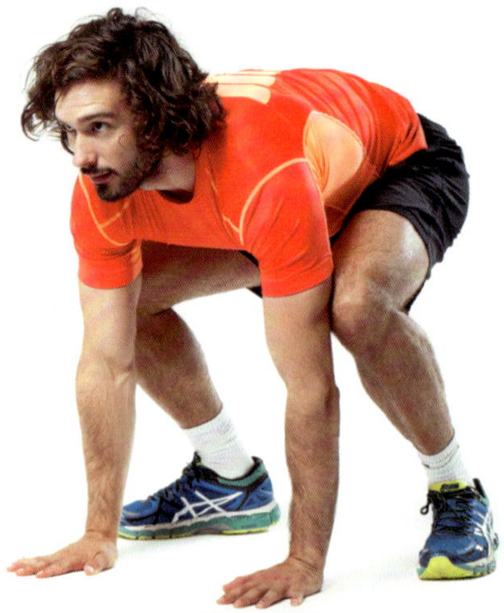

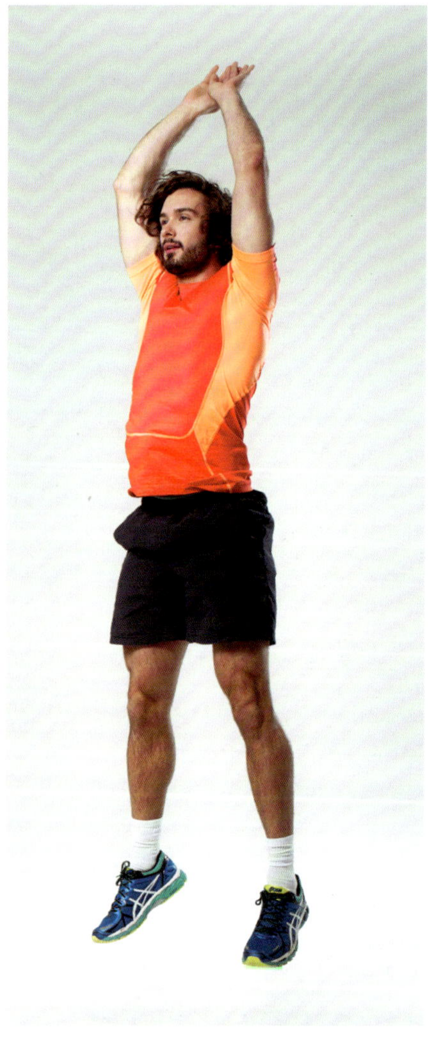

Cool down

Cooling down is really important for your muscles and joints. Have a slow walk or cycle to let your heart rate return to normal. Static stretching or foam rolling can really help reduce your muscle soreness. You may find you experience DOMS (Delayed Onset Muscle Soreness) after your first few sessions. This is totally normal and lasts between 24 and 72 hours. Don't worry, it will pass. It's just your body's way of letting you know you've worked hard, and it will reward you by growing stronger and leaner.

When do I do it?

HIIT cardio is effective at any time of day, so I always recommend doing it when you have the most energy. This could be in the morning before work or late in the evening. Remember, this is your time to 'earn' your post-workout carbs.

How often do I do it?

You should aim to do HIIT 4 or 5 days a week for maximum results. If you can't manage that many workouts each week, that's fine – just do what you can and keep a good routine. Remember, though, that on rest days you will be consuming 3 meals from the reduced-carbohydrate menu, so if you want to enjoy your carbs, then you are going to need to find time to smash out a quick HIIT.

Good luck with your workouts. Remember to push yourself and aim to progress each week: this could mean going 0.5km/h faster each week on the treadmill or increasing the weight of your dumbbells by 1kg each week. With progression comes strength, and a strong lean body is exactly what you will earn. Be patient and be consistent. Rome wasn't built in a day.

> **'Be patient and be consistent'**

WORKOUT 2: *RESISTANCE HIIT*

This full-body workout is going to take a bit longer than the HIIT cardio one, as it's going to focus not only on elevating your heart rate, but also on increasing lean muscle with resistance training. By increasing your lean muscle mass, you will increase your metabolic rate, which means you will burn even more fat and can enjoy more food as you get leaner.

All you will need for this is a set of dumbbells for added resistance and an exercise mat. If you are a beginner, start with light weights and aim to increase them as you get stronger. You are going to do the following exercises in a circuit and perform as many reps as possible in 30 seconds. You will then rest for 45 seconds between each exercise. As you get fitter and stronger, you can reduce the rest time to 30 seconds or increase the total number of rounds of 5 full circuits.

1. **Press-ups with dumbbell row**
2. **Dumbbell squats**
3. **Shoulder presses**
4. **Dumbbell lunges**
5. **Bicep curls**

1. 30 seconds Press-ups with dumbbell row

(You can do these on your knees if you prefer.)

45 seconds rest

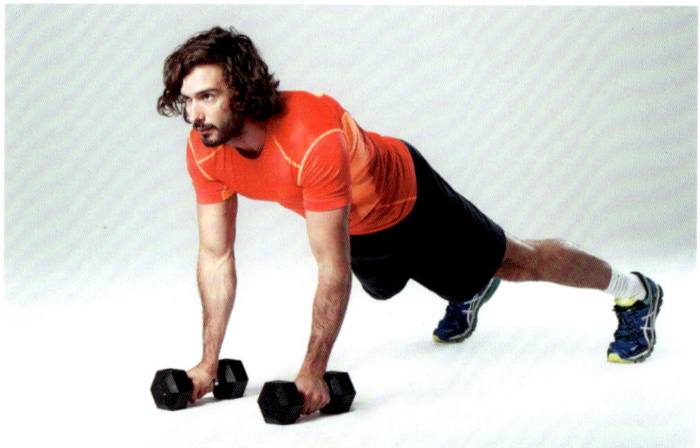

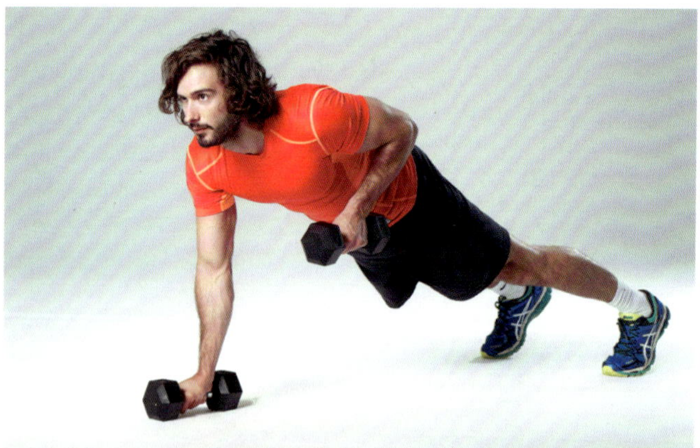

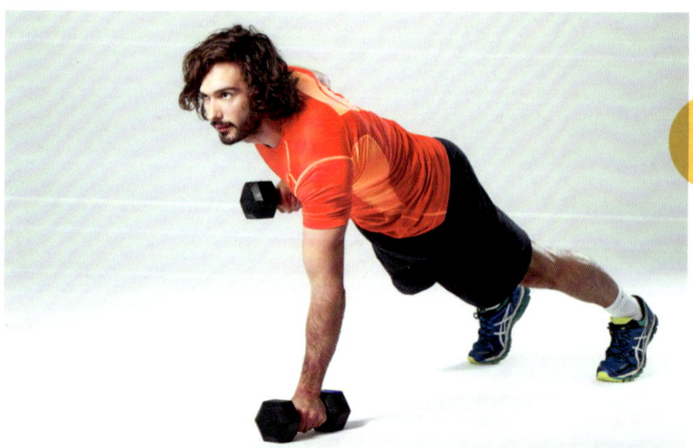

2. 30 seconds
Dumbbell squats
45 seconds rest

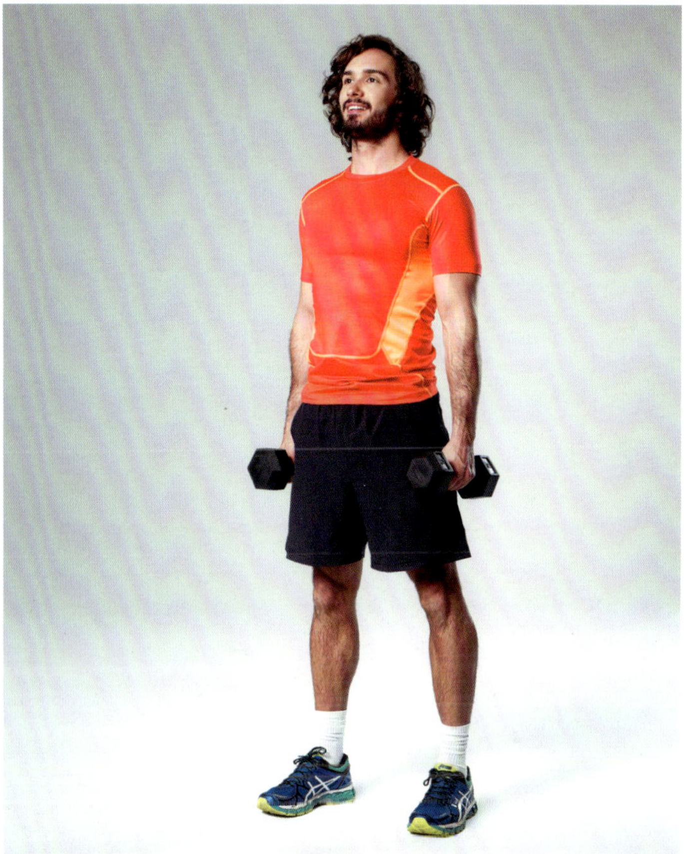

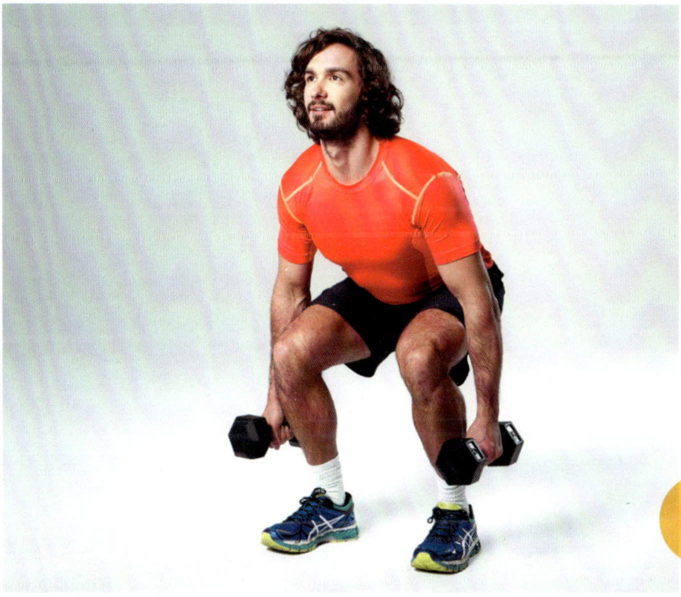

3. **30 seconds Shoulder presses**

45 seconds rest

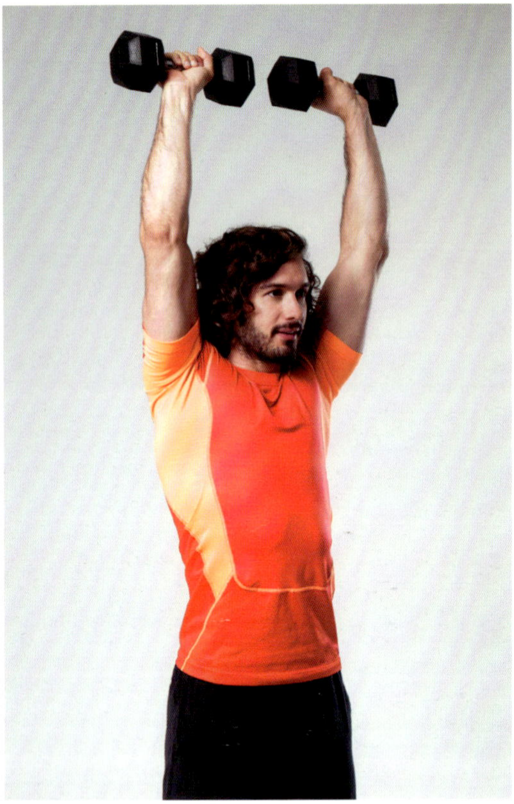

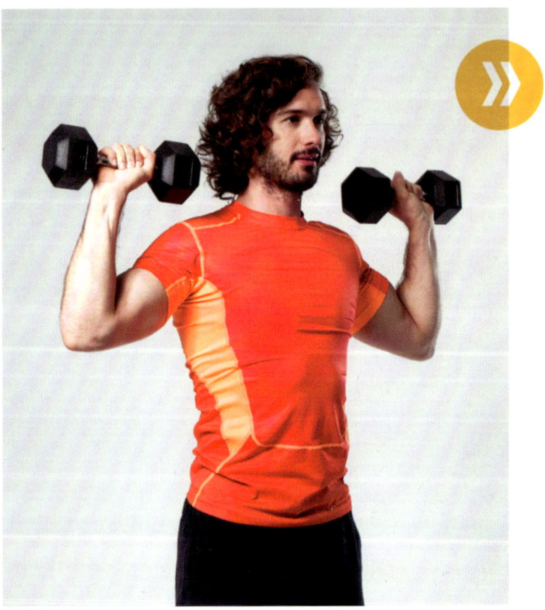

4. **30 seconds Dumbbell lunges**

45 seconds rest

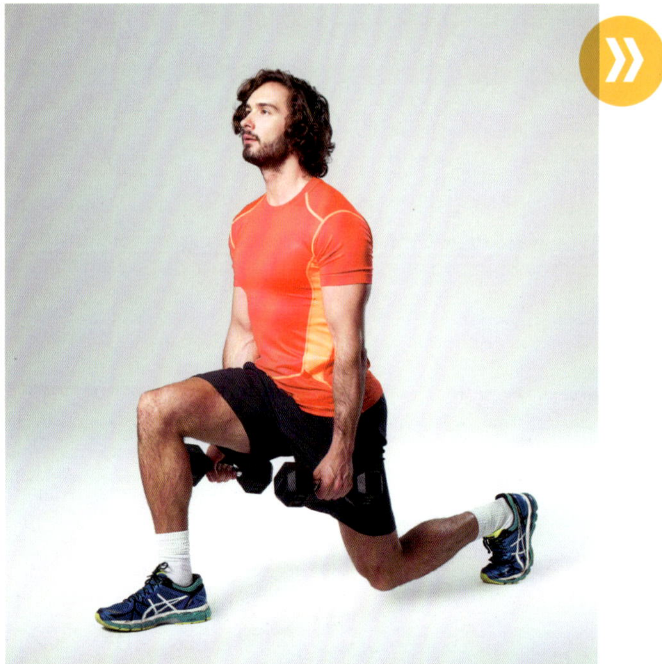

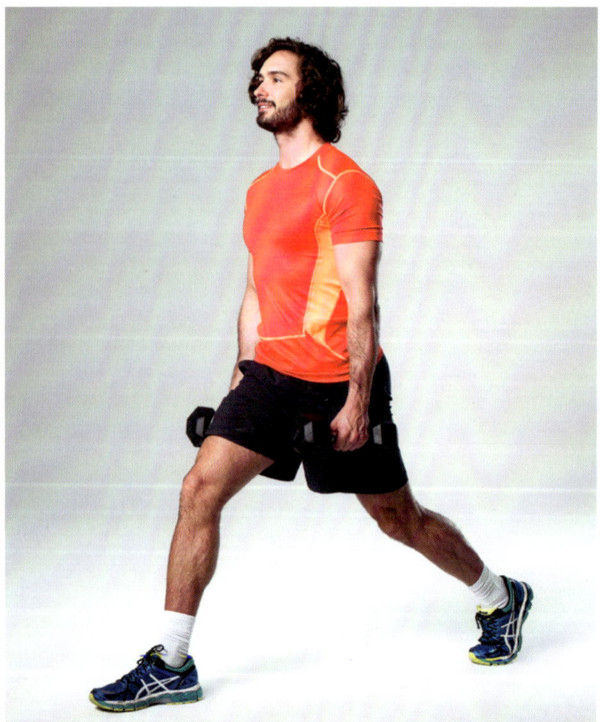

5. **30 seconds**

Bicep curls

45 seconds rest

Repeat this circuit 3–5 times depending on your fitness level (approximately 30 minutes).

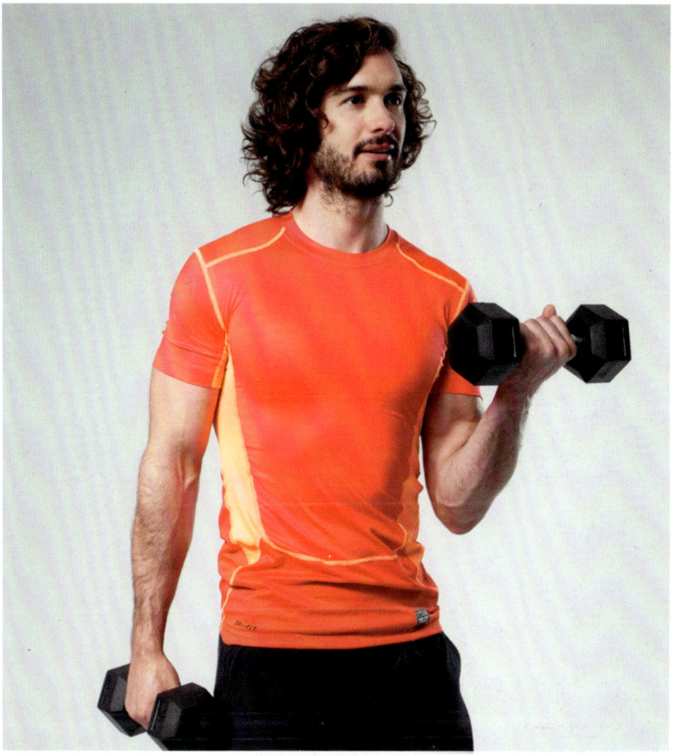

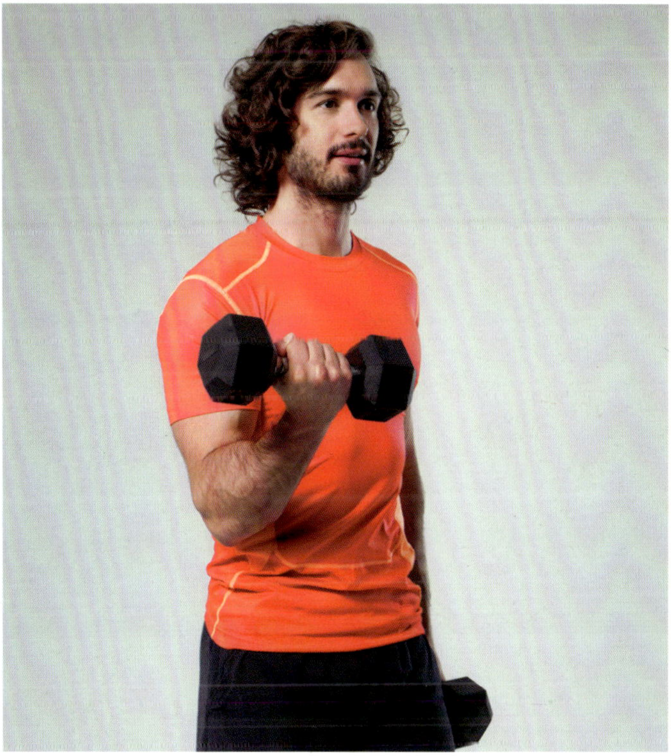

7

RESULTS: MY LEAN WINNERS

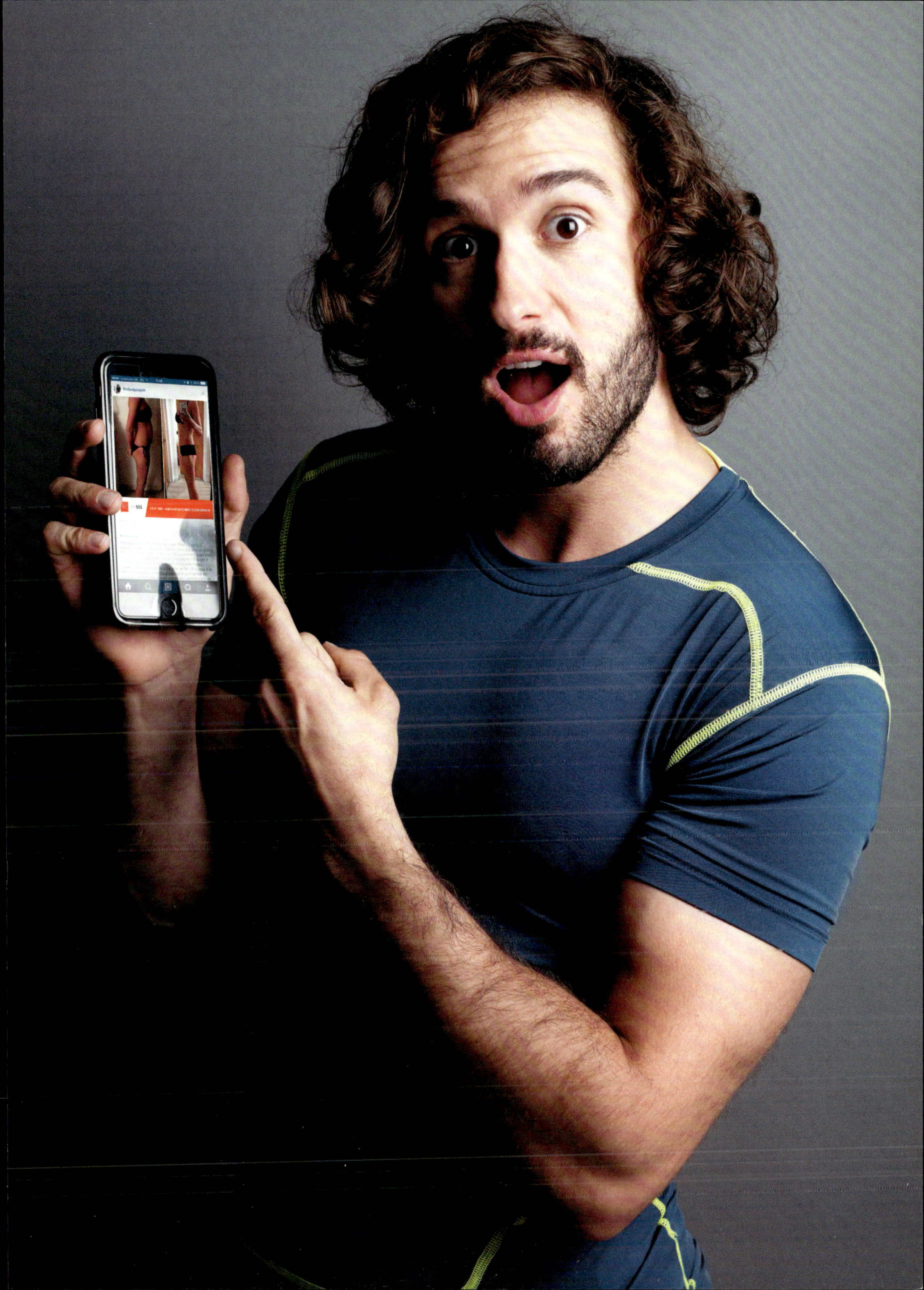

MY LEAN WINNERS

For me, one of the most rewarding things about the 90 Day Shift, Shape and Sustain plan is seeing the incredible transformations of my clients, and reading their testimonials. I call them my lean winners – and, although I never actually get to meet them, I'm proud of them all. Not everyone wants to share their stories online and most of those who do want to remain anonymous, but their progress pictures really inspire people. The daily transformations I post on Instagram are one of the reasons so many people have signed up to the plan.

There's nothing better than seeing people of all ages, shapes and sizes succeed in their goals. Often many of them have battled with their weight for years on diets, but in 90 days they transform their body and their relationship with food forever. Knowing that I have educated someone and improved their health and self-confidence is what inspires me to work even harder to help more people. My plan isn't all about weight loss. I have helped people with IBS (irritable bowel syndrome), diabetes, underactive thyroid glands, PCOS (polycystic ovary syndrome) and many other conditions to improve their way of life.

I could fill a whole book with transformations and my graduate heroes, but unfortunately I can only include a handful here. To see more lean winners, visit thebodycoach.co.uk and check out the Transformations gallery, where you'll find thousands of inspirational people, all winning their own little battles and getting fitter and stronger.

Here are just a few of the transformations from the plan (for privacy reasons, I have not included faces or @names), showing some 4-week, 8-week and 12-week transformations, to give you a better idea of the results achieved.

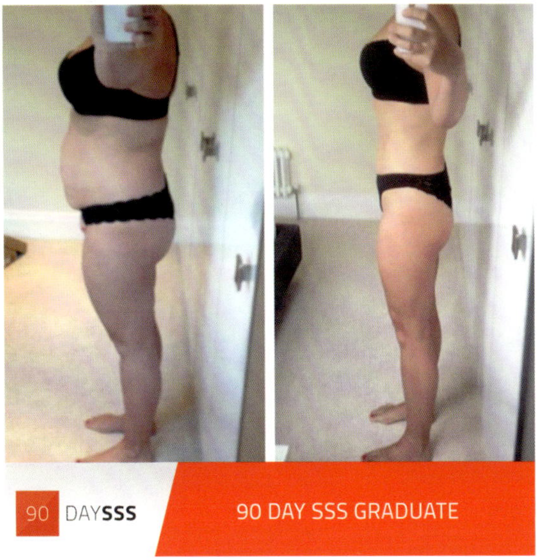

★

'The 90 Day SSS plan has changed my life. The education I have received has been invaluable, and I can't recommend this plan enough! I finally feel in control of my diet and my training. I LOVE the gym, and I love the feeling of being full and satisfied from nutritious healthy food. I feel immensely proud, and will be celebrating with a treat tonight before getting right back on that wagon and back in the gym in the morning!!! This is me now: fit, healthy and happy.' **Sarah**

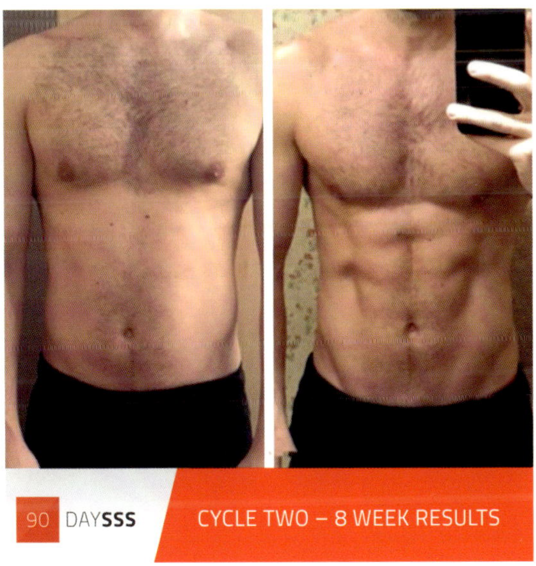

★

'The amount of food was unbelievable. It took a while to get used to it, but once I got the hang of it, it was so simple. My body shape is still changing for the better, and I'm so happy with it. I am so much stronger and feel great!' **Jason**

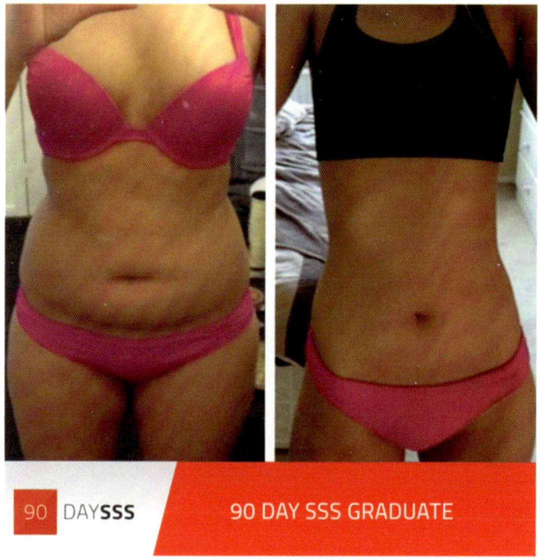

★

'I cannot believe the #90daysssplan is already over – it's absolutely flown by. To say I'm extremely pleased with the progress is an understatement! Towards the end of last year I hit a real low. I hated my body and the way I looked, and finally decided to pluck up the courage and do something about it. Life did throw me a few curve balls during cycle 3, so I haven't been able to follow the plan 100%, but I always tried to make up for it the following day with an extra-hard HIIT session. I've done all my workouts from home, so there really are no excuses! Thank you for giving me the confidence I never had.' **Kerry**

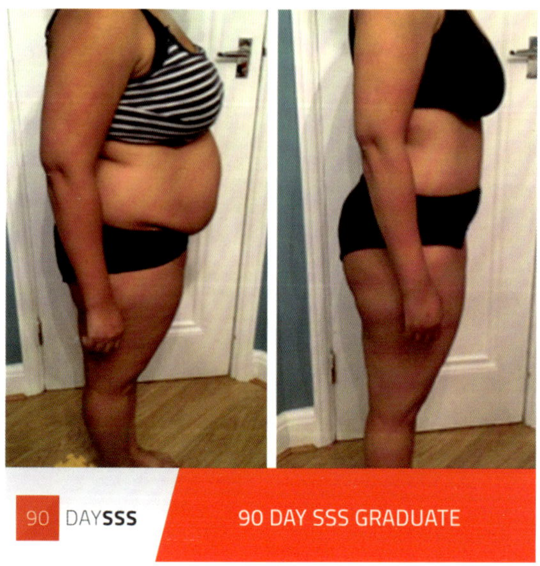

★

'I'm so happy that I decided to contact Joe. He has honestly changed my life. I really had zero confidence after having children, but since being on the plan not only has my confidence increased ten-fold, it has pushed me to do things in my life that I would have previously been scared to do. Because I'm feeling better, the relationships around me are more positive, and I can play with my children without getting tired. I feel motivated to carry on. The help from Joe has been invaluable and also the kind words from others doing the plan on social media. What he's telling others about healthy fats and body image is so incredibly important, regardless of whether you want to lose weight, gain weight or just get healthy – Joe's plan is a way of life, and the energy and passion behind it make you want to listen. I've even put my scales away. Thank you so much, Joe!' **Jihan**

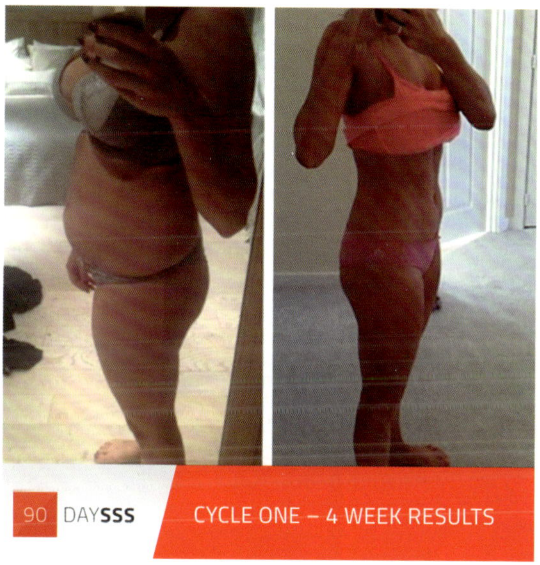

★

'I signed up to the #90daysssplan after seeing the amazing results one of my friends had. I have done every diet you can imagine, but have never seen results like those I got with The Body Coach. I really, really love food and love big portions, so every diet I have ever tried, I have struggled with hunger and cravings, but not on this one. I couldn't quite get my head around how I could eat this much and still lose weight, as I have always thought the less you eat the more you lose. The workouts are tough, but they are only about 25 minutes long, so easy enough to get through. In cycle one I tended to do them at home, following YouTube videos or using an interval timer app – which literally meant that after 25 minutes I was all done and could enjoy my yummy meal.' **Sophie**

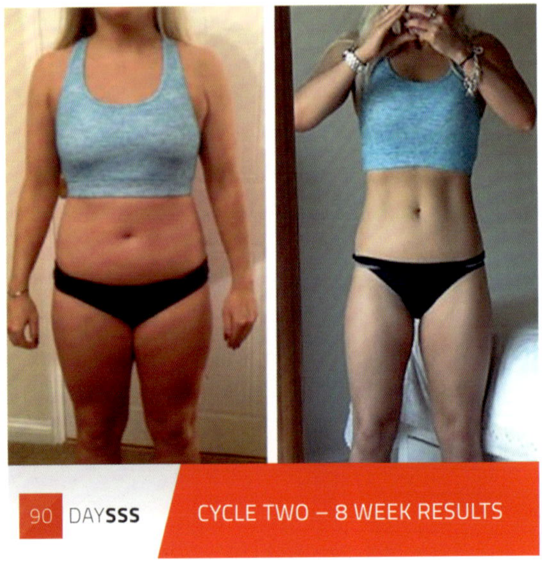

★

'The workouts are brilliant – I loved mixing HIIT and using weights, and I could feel myself getting stronger each week. Although I haven't stuck to the food side of things as well as I could have, due to being on Easter holidays, having a few boozy nights out and going away for 5 days, I can honestly say I haven't missed a workout!' **Sarah**

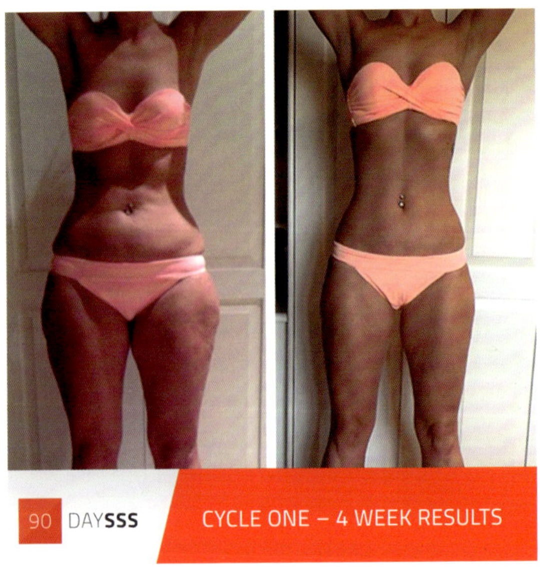

★

'I started following Joe on Instagram and signed up straight away when I saw all the amazing transformation photos. For years I have tried every single low calorie diet and have always been unhappy with my body, especially my tree trunk legs, and was obsessed with the sad step! After seeing my own transformation photo I was shocked that the "tree trunks" had finally started to shrink. I never thought they would as I always assumed I was just a big-legged girl and no matter what exercise I did or what low-calorie diet I was on, my legs would just stay the same! Considering I used to be obsessed with weighing myself daily, after seeing my photo I think it's amazing that I actually weigh exactly the same as when I started but have lost a whole 10 inches from my body. I definitely will never be obsessed again with what the sad step has to say! I did have a few cheat days, but I stuck to the HIIT sessions 100% which I really enjoyed and can't wait to introduce the weights in cycle 2!' **Rhonda**

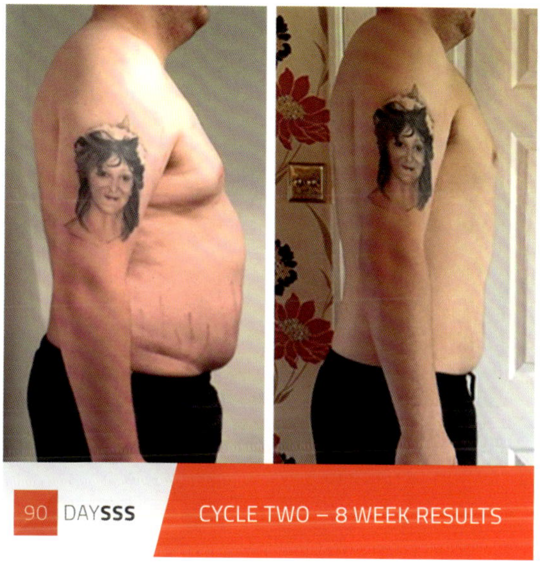

★

'For months, even years, I never gave a thought to the food I would eat – and this, combined with no exercise at all and obviously getting older, took a massive toll on my body. Around Christmas last year I looked in the mirror and just realized I really needed to do something. I found Joe purely through chance, with a friend liking one of his videos. I then investigated further and liked the way Joe incorporated humour into fitness and nutrition. This, coupled with the results, made me take the plunge and sign up to the #90daysssplan. Having a complete lack of fitness, I found the first weeks of HIIT tough – I knew I would – but my own determination to plough on, and the support from The Body Coach team, pushed me through. Soon after, I was finding I was enjoying sweating like an absolute beast at 6am . . . strange, I know! Incorporating the weights into cycle two for me was totally alien, having never used weights before! Preparation is most definitely key. I spend around 2 hours in the kitchen on a Sunday, and this sets me up for the week.' **Danny**

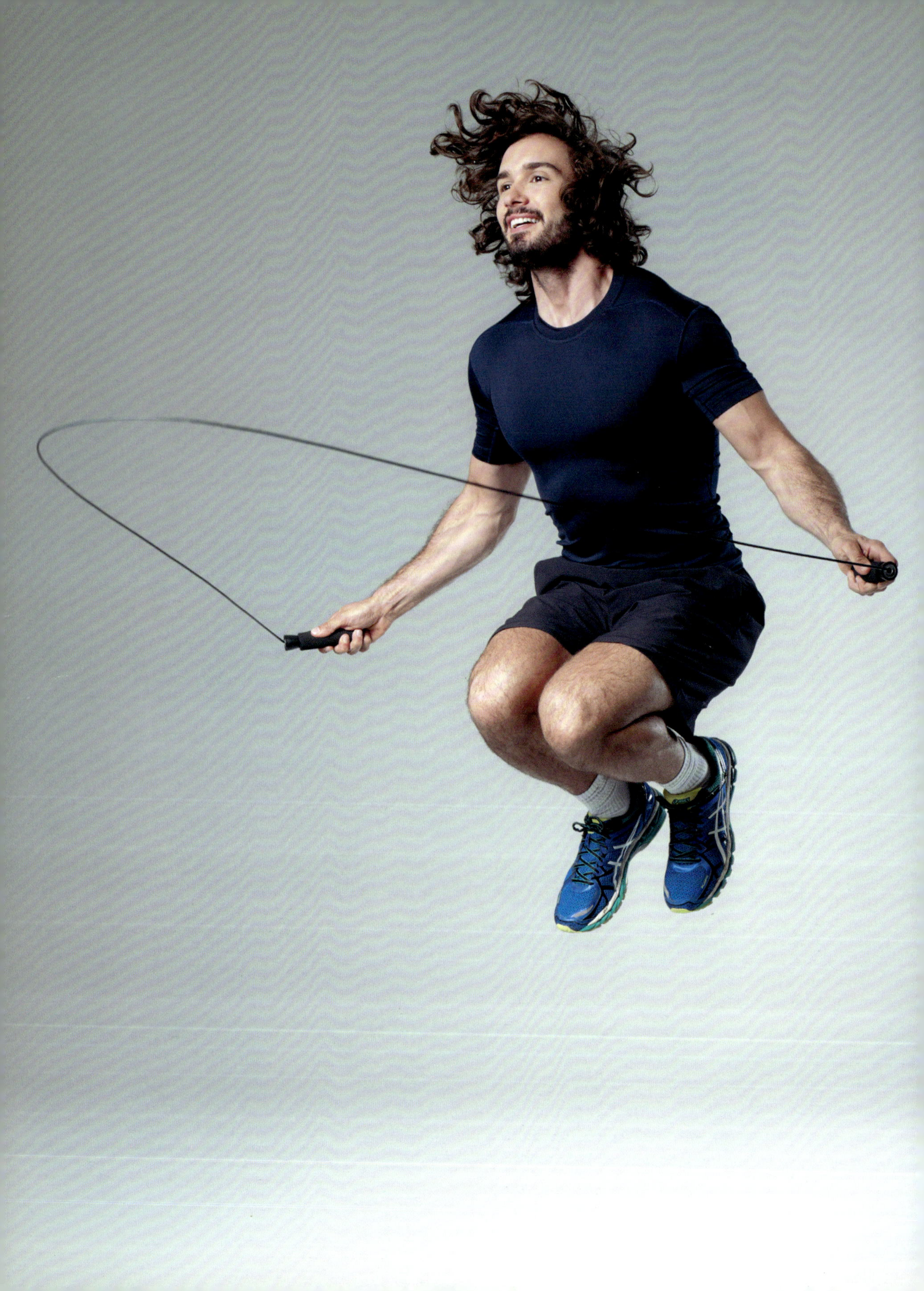

MY TYPICAL WEEK

I thought it would be useful to show you how I eat in a typical week, to give you ideas for your own meal planning. You'll notice I eat some of the same meals more than once a week, as I like to batch-cook and keep meals in the fridge for when I'm busy. This really helps me stay on track, as I'm far less likely to grab junk food on the go when I know I have my meals waiting at home when I get in.

You'll also notice that I always have a protein shake with honey immediately after I train. The glucose elevates my blood sugar levels post-workout, triggering the release of insulin, which will send protein to my muscles and start repairing them. When I have a protein shake as a snack at any other time of the day, I don't add honey, but just mix a scoop of protein with some ice and water.

I usually eat my post-workout meal about an hour after I finish a workout, but you can eat sooner or later if you prefer. No matter how early or late you train, you must always choose a carbohydrate-refuel meal after your workout. This is the time your muscles really need to be topped up with glycogen and fed protein to build and repair muscle tissue.

You may think I'm a bit odd eating burgers or stir-fries for breakfast, but I'm giving my body exactly what it needs to burn fat and build lean muscle. Once you start to think outside the cereal box and get over the idea of eating what feels like dinner at breakfast, you'll soon get used to it. Your work colleagues may think you're mad pulling out a chicken stir-fry at 9am, but while they're eating their sugary cereal and gaining body fat, you'll be winning and burning body fat.

The most important thing is to make your meal plan suit your lifestyle, so be flexible in your approach. As long as you consume your 3 meals and 2 snacks at some point during the day, you will burn fat and build lean muscle.

JOE'S PROTEIN SHAKE

1 scoop (30g) vanilla protein powder
15g honey
100g baby spinach leaves
handful of ice cubes

METHOD

Throw everything in the blender with a good splash of water and blitz until smooth.

	MONDAY	TUESDAY	WEDNESDAY	THURSDAY	FRIDAY	SATURDAY	SUNDAY
Training: am	7am Cardio HIIT		7am Resistance HIIT		7am Resistance HIIT	Rest day	Rest day
Post workout	Joe's protein shake		Joe's protein shake		Joe's protein shake		
Meal 1	Build-up bagel	Poached salmon with bacon	Protein pancakes	Griddled midget trees and spears with eggs	Bad-boy burrito	Griddled midget trees and spears with eggs	Cinnamon reduced-carb oatmeal
Snack	30g nuts	Apple	Avocado ranch dip	75g blueberries	Whipped-up herby cream cheese with celery	30g nuts	Protein shake
Meal 2	Lamb koftas with Greek salad	Turkey meatballs with feta	Goan fish curry	Asian duck salad	Turkey mince lettuce boats	Joe's chicken pie	Thai green chicken curry
Snack	Protein shake	Tuna and courgette fritters	30g nuts	Protein shake	30g nuts	Whipped-up herby cream cheese with celery	Protein cupcakes
Training pm		6pm Cardio HIIT		6pm Cardio HIIT		Rest day	Rest day
Post workout		Joe's protein shake		Joe's protein shake			
Meal 3	Teriyaki salmon with courgette noodles	Thai beef stir-fry	Sea bass with spiced cauliflower, peas and paneer	In-a-hurry curry fried rice	Joe's chicken pie	Eat out*	Lamb koftas with Greek salad

*Keeping it lean when eating out

One of my favourite things in the world is eating out with family and friends. I have a very simple philosophy when it comes to 'cheat' meals. If I know I am going to go for a blow-out meal, then I like to earn it beforehand with a quick 20-minute HIIT session, so I can enjoy the extra carbs and treats as my refuel meal. If I go out for a meal when I haven't trained, then I try to stick to just fats and proteins and leave the carbs alone, opting for something like grilled steak or fish with lots of vegetables and a big drizzle of olive oil. These small food choices really will make a big difference over time and allow you to stay lean.

	MONDAY	TUESDAY	WEDNESDAY	THURSDAY	FRIDAY	SATURDAY	SUNDAY
Training: am							
Post workout							
Meal 1							
Snack							
Meal 2							
Snack							
Training pm							
Post workout							
Meal 3							

USE THIS TABLE TO PLAN YOUR OWN MEALS AND WORKOUTS FOR THE WEEK

Prepping like a boss

I hope you love the food in this book as much as I do, and get inspired to start cooking more and prepping like a boss so you can achieve the healthy body you want. Just remember that fat loss takes time, dedication and consistency. You can and will get lean – just keep working hard and make it a habit to eat the Lean in 15 way.

LEAN IN 15 HEROES

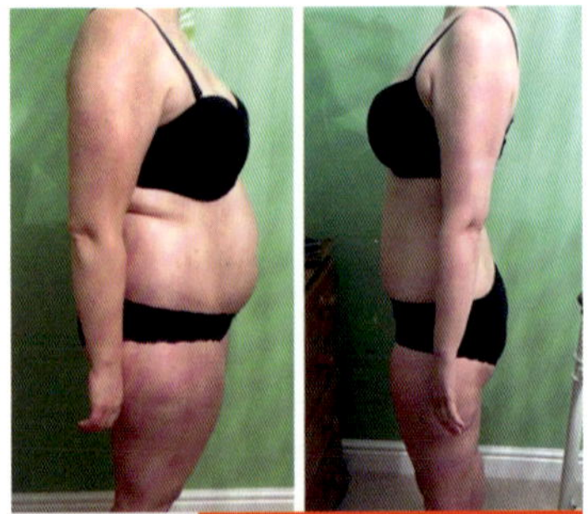
90 DAYSSS — 90 DAY SSS GRADUATE

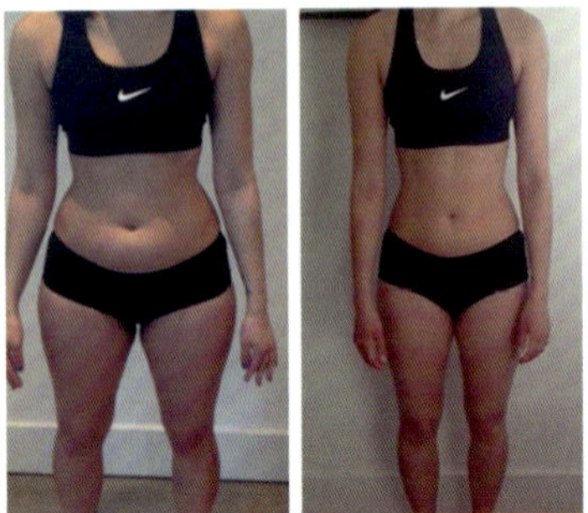
90 DAYSSS — 90 DAY SSS GRADUATE

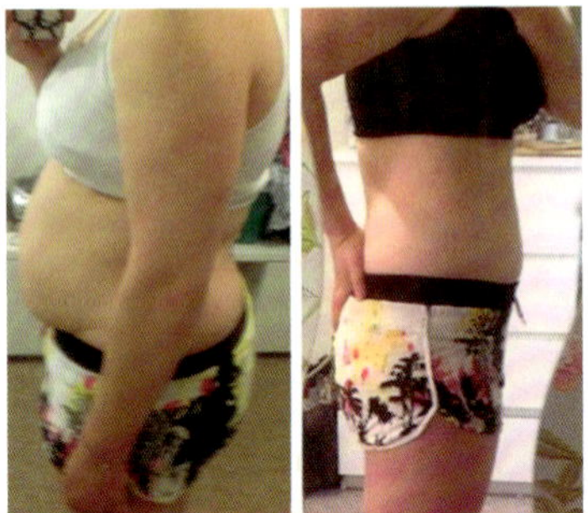
90 DAYSSS — CYCLE ONE – 4 WEEK RESULTS

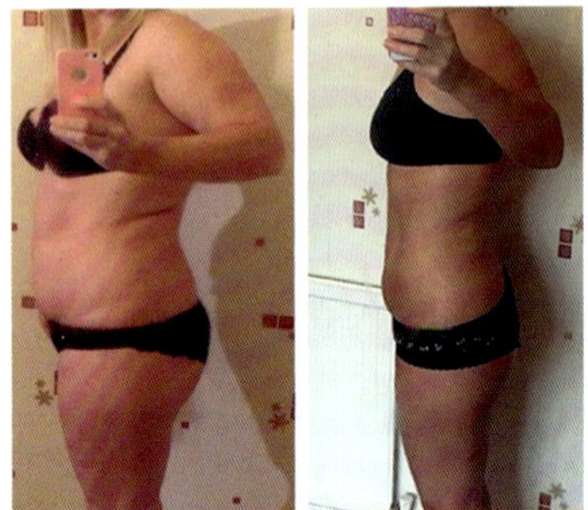
90 DAYSSS — CYCLE TWO – 8 WEEK RESULTS

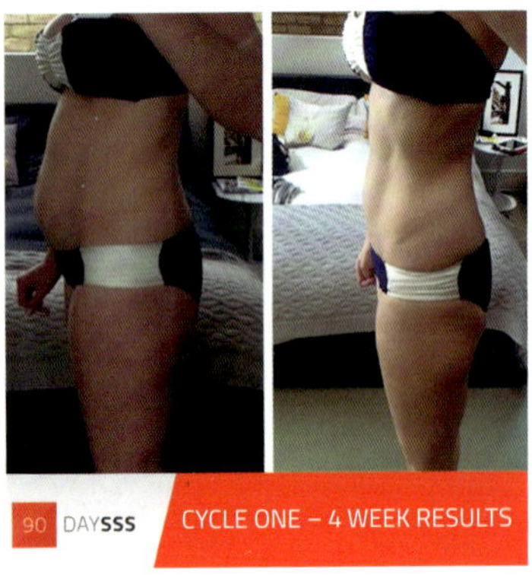
90 DAYSSS — CYCLE ONE – 4 WEEK RESULTS

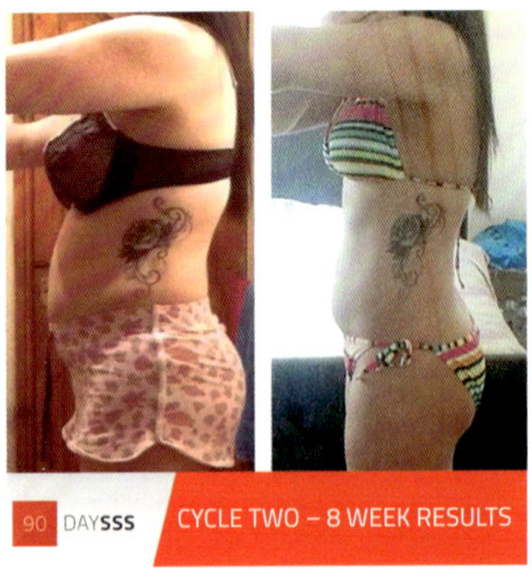
90 DAYSSS — CYCLE TWO – 8 WEEK RESULTS

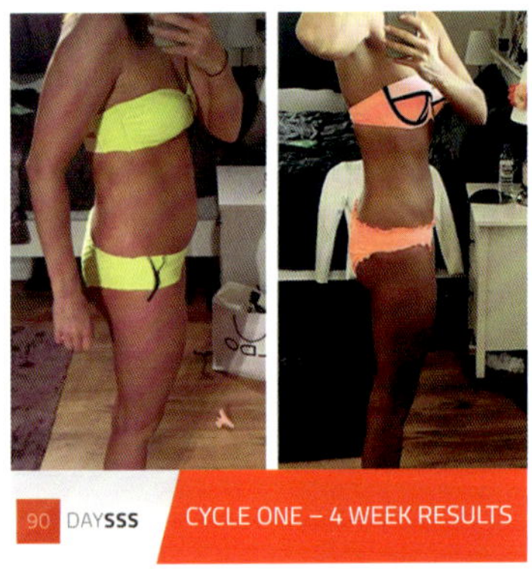
90 DAYSSS — CYCLE ONE – 4 WEEK RESULTS

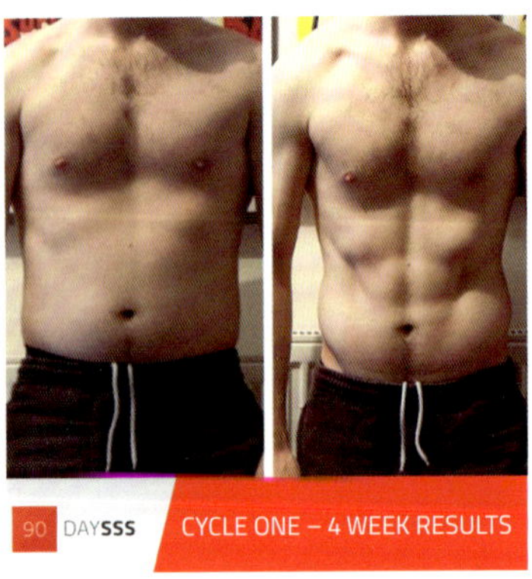
90 DAYSSS — CYCLE ONE – 4 WEEK RESULTS

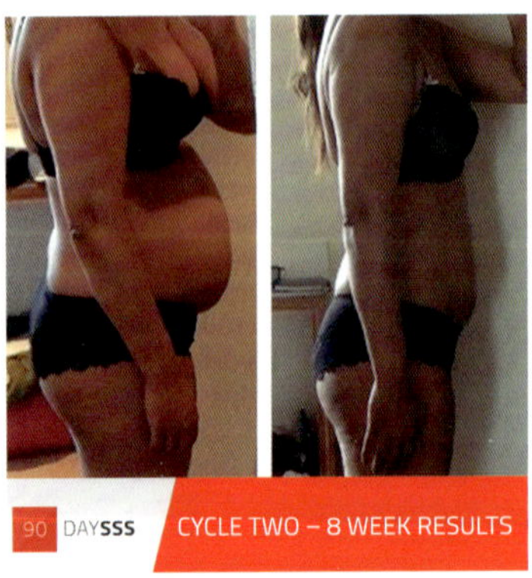
90 DAYSSS — CYCLE TWO – 8 WEEK RESULTS

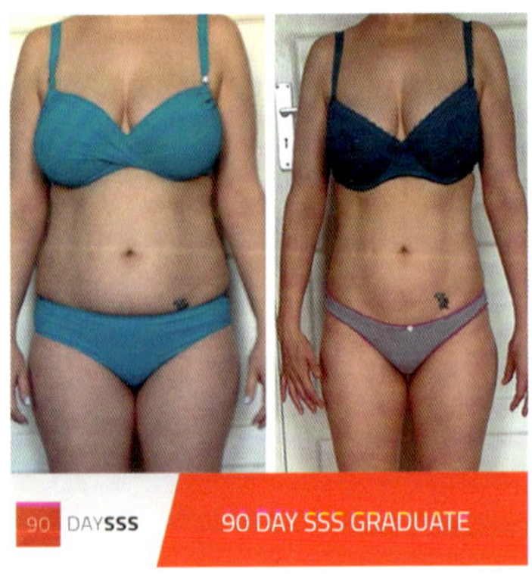
90 DAYSSS — 90 DAY SSS GRADUATE

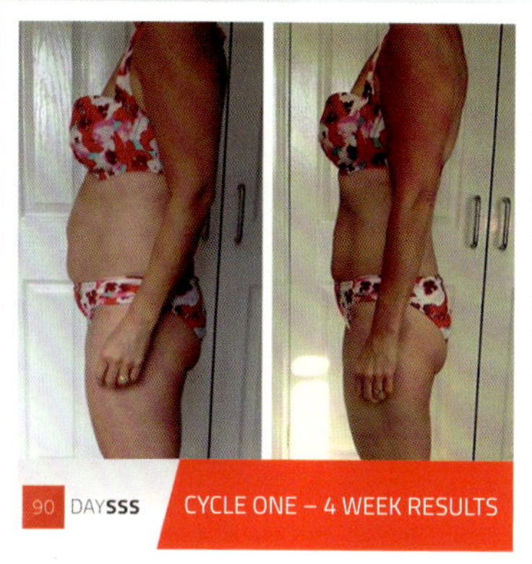
90 DAYSSS
CYCLE ONE – 4 WEEK RESULTS

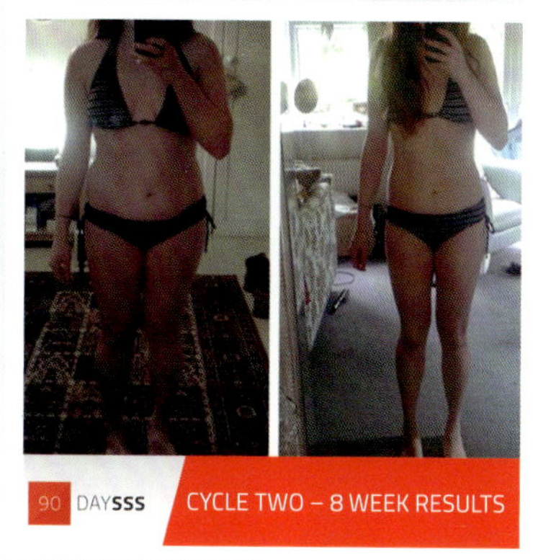
90 DAYSSS
CYCLE TWO – 8 WEEK RESULTS

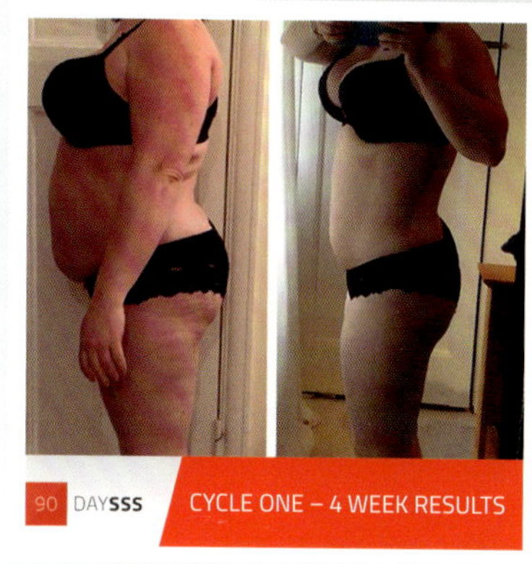
90 DAYSSS
CYCLE ONE – 4 WEEK RESULTS

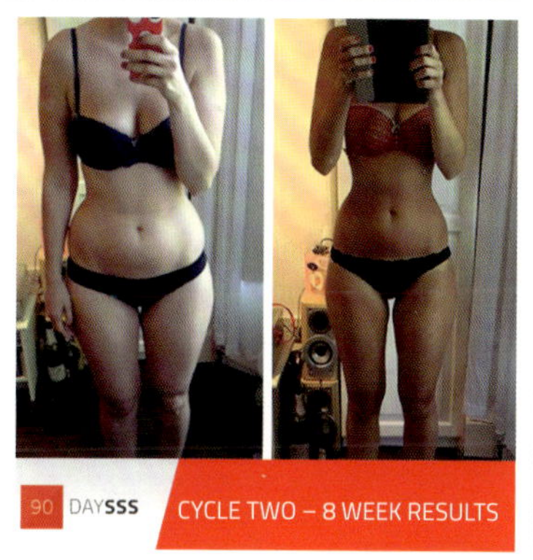
90 DAYSSS
CYCLE TWO – 8 WEEK RESULTS

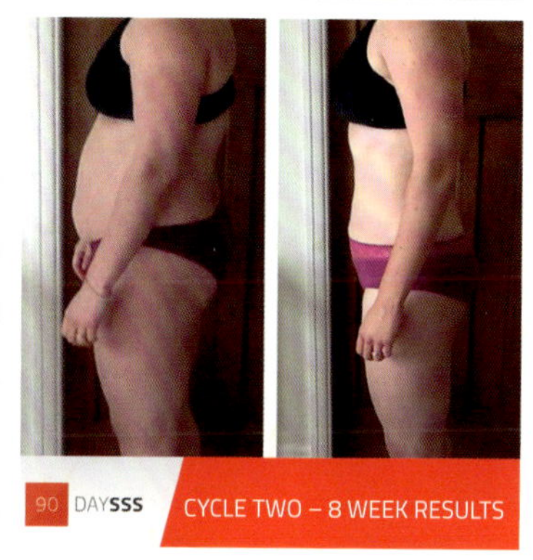
90 DAYSSS
CYCLE TWO – 8 WEEK RESULTS

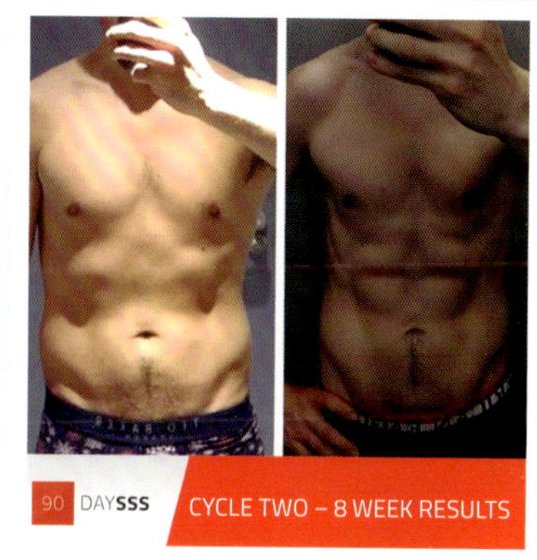
90 DAYSSS
CYCLE TWO – 8 WEEK RESULTS

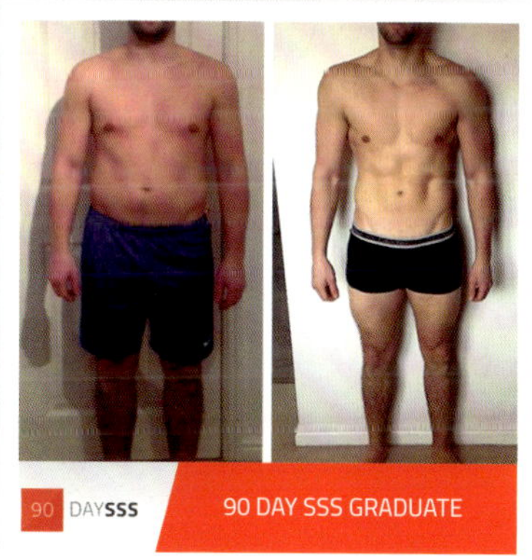
90 DAYSSS
90 DAY SSS GRADUATE

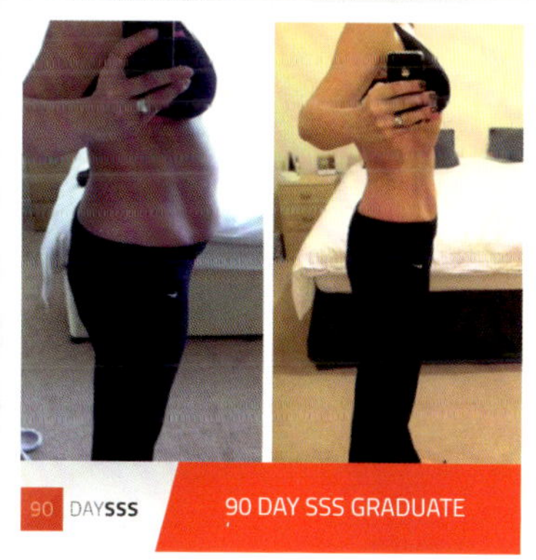
90 DAYSSS
90 DAY SSS GRADUATE

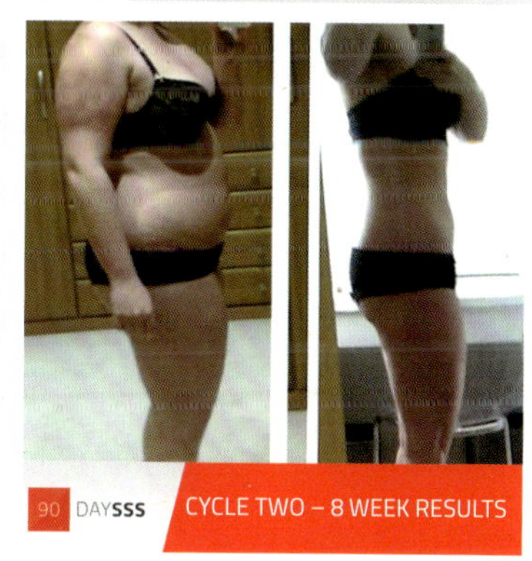
90 DAYSSS
CYCLE TWO – 8 WEEK RESULTS

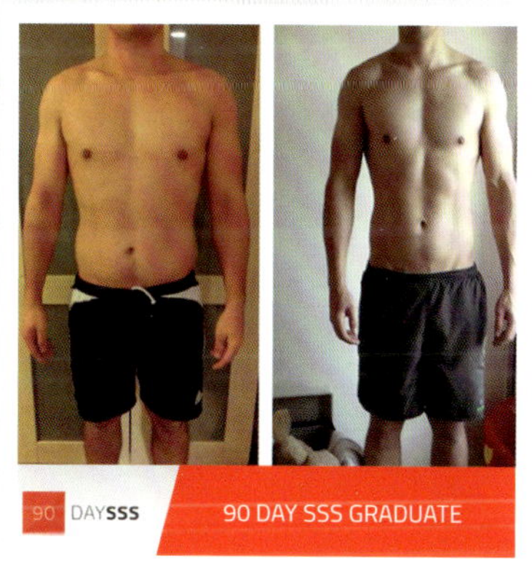
90 DAYSSS
90 DAY SSS GRADUATE

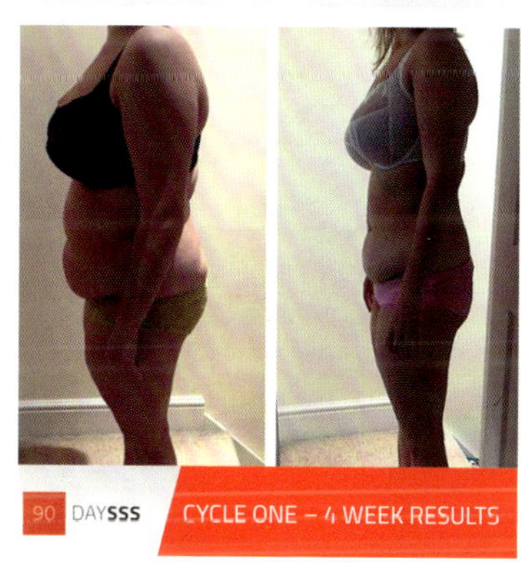
90 DAYSSS
CYCLE ONE – 4 WEEK RESULTS

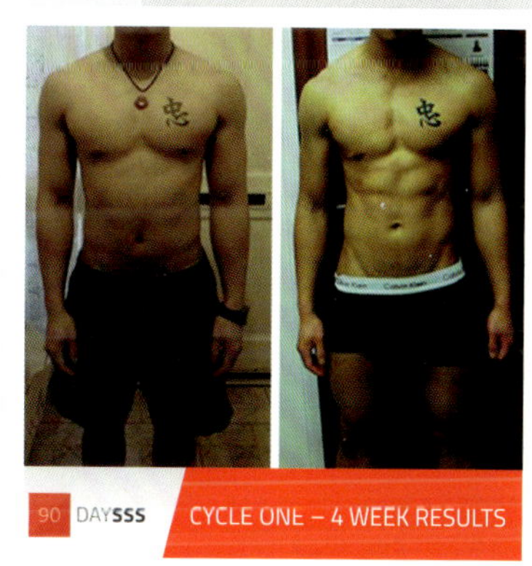
90 DAYSSS
CYCLE ONE – 4 WEEK RESULTS

INDEX

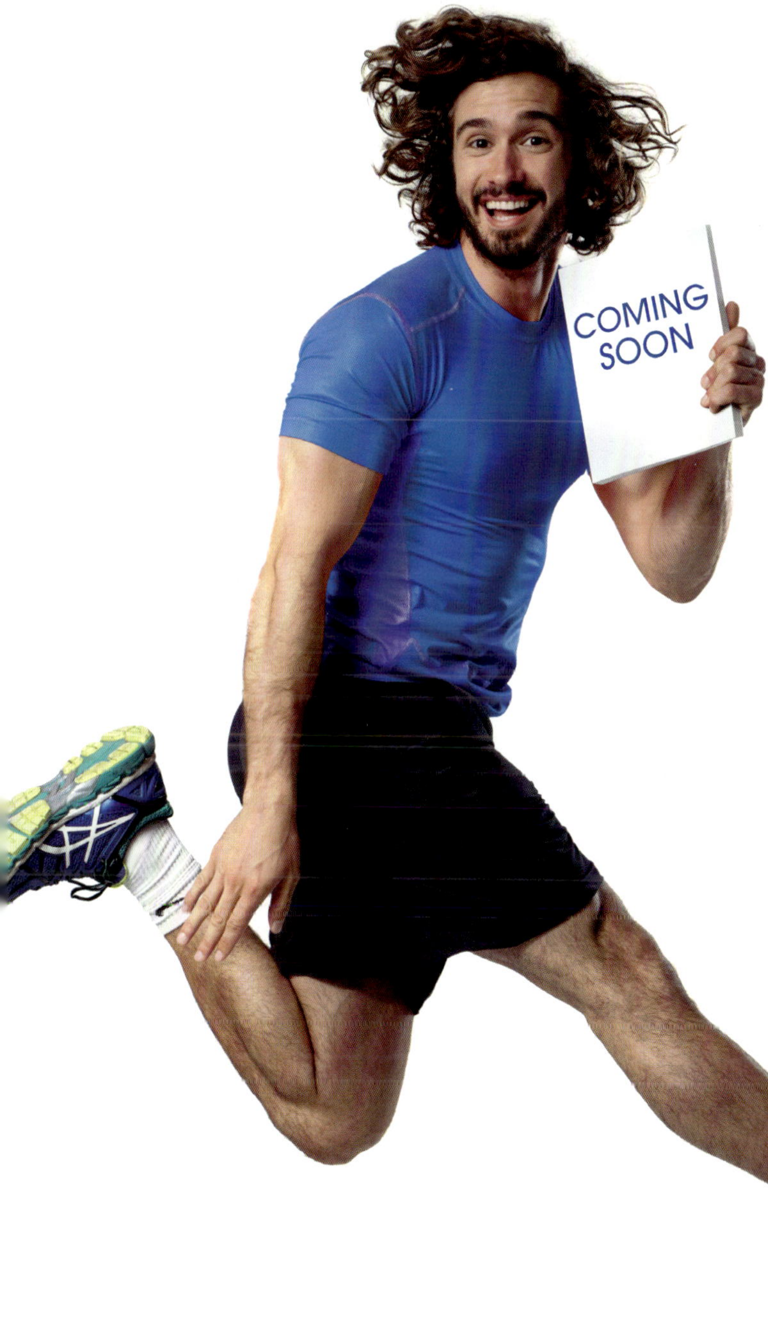

ACKNOWLEDGEMENTS

I would like to start by thanking everyone who has ever completed my 90 Day plan and followed me on social media. Because of you, I've been able to build a following, spread my message and have the opportunity to release this book. Without you, I would just have been a dude in a kitchen talking to midget trees, so thanks for sticking around and sharing my videos with others.

I would also like to say thank you to all my friends and family who love and support me in my goals.

See you in June for *Lean in 15*, volume 2 – *The Shape Plan*.

CREDITS

Publisher: Carole Tonkinson
Assistant Editor: Olivia Morris
Design: Ami Smithson
Desk Editor: Claire Gatzen
Food Photography: Maja Smend
Fitness Photography: Glen Burrows
Food Styling: Bianca Nice
Prop Styling: Lydia Brun
Make-up Artist: Jo McKenna

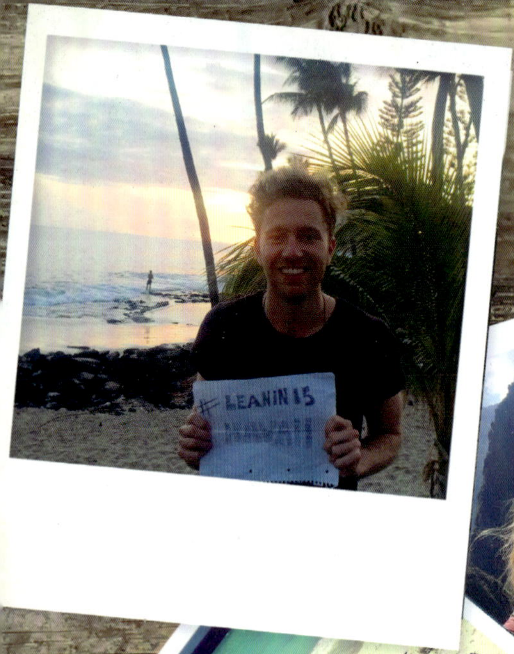

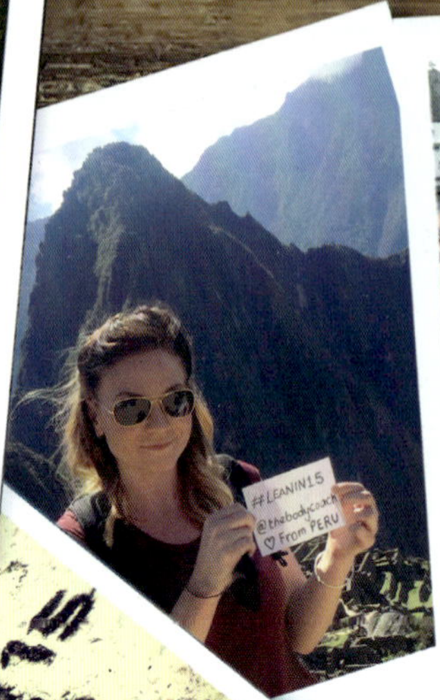

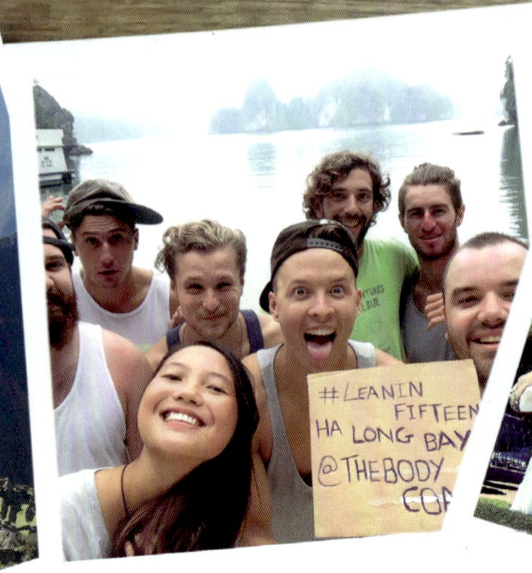

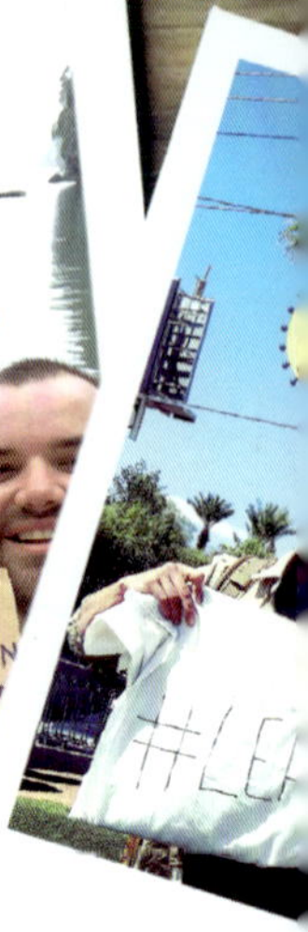

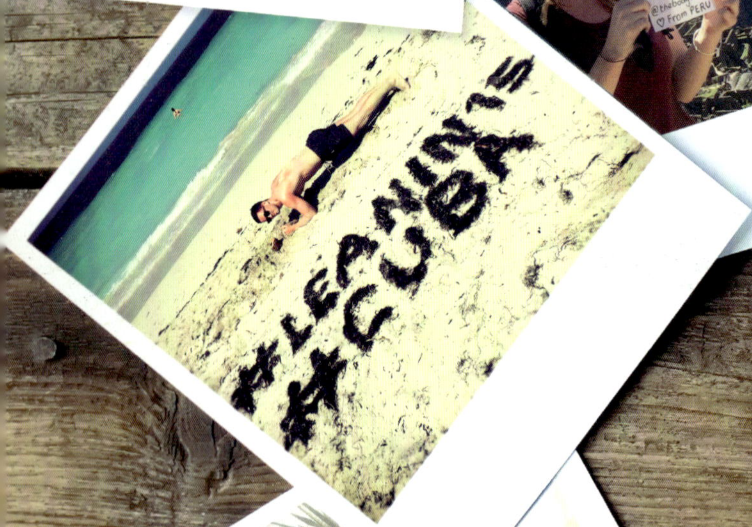

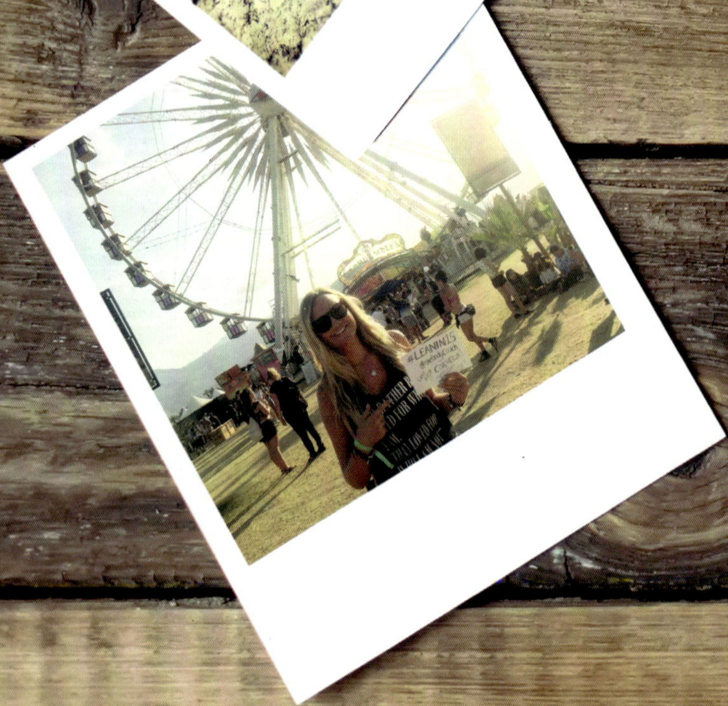

LEAN IN 15 AROUND THE WORLD

Tag your own pictures from around the world with the hashtag #Leanin15

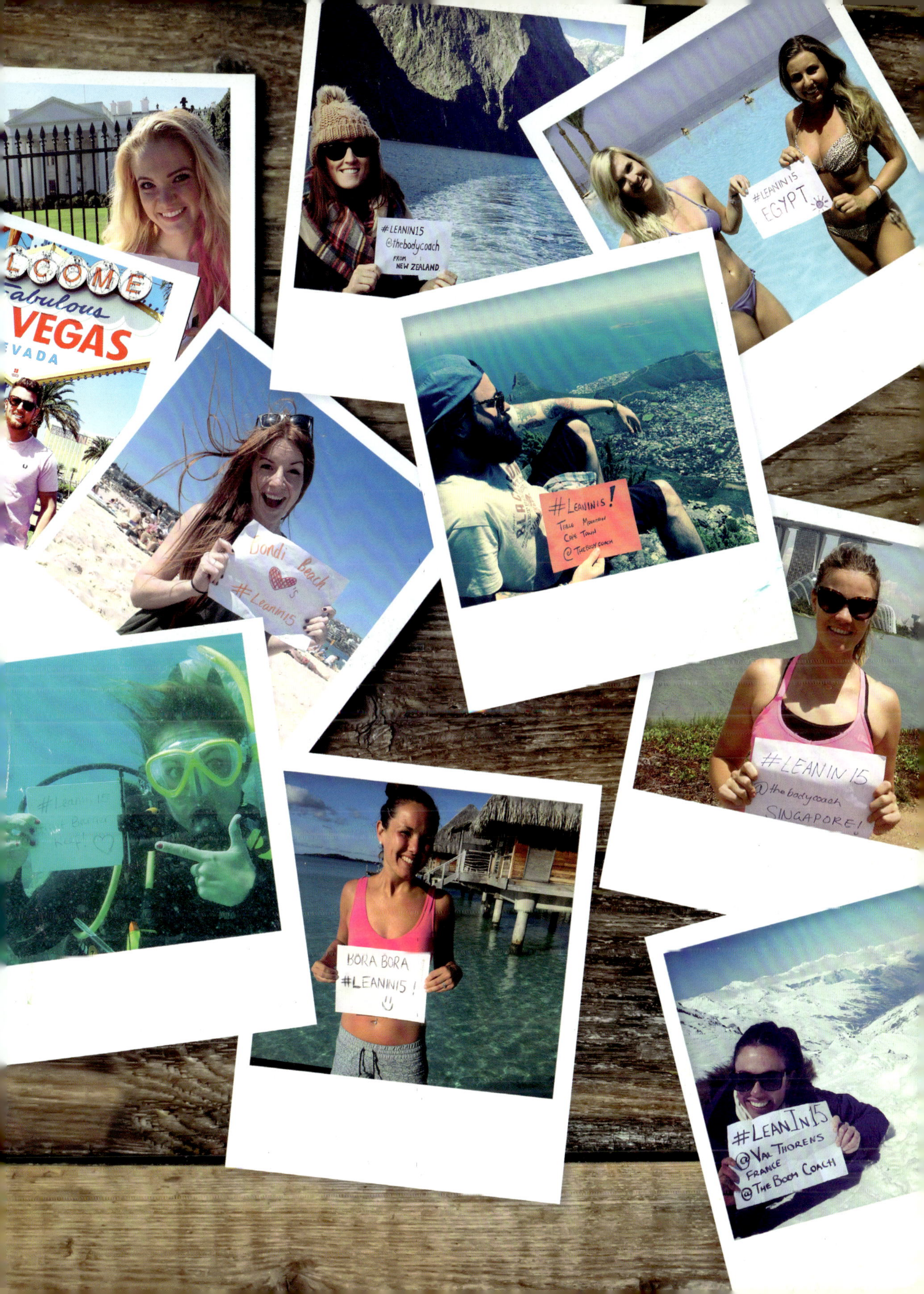

LCOME
Fabulous
VEGAS
EVADA
#LEANIN15
@thebodycoach
FROM NEW ZEALAND
#LEANIN15
EGYPT
#LEANIN15!
Table Mountain
Cape Town
@ THEBODYCOACH
Bondi Beach
's
#Leanin15
#LEANIN 15
@thebodycoach
SINGAPORE!
BORA BORA
#LEANIN15!
#LEANIn15
@ VAL THORENS
FRANCE
@ THE BODY COACH

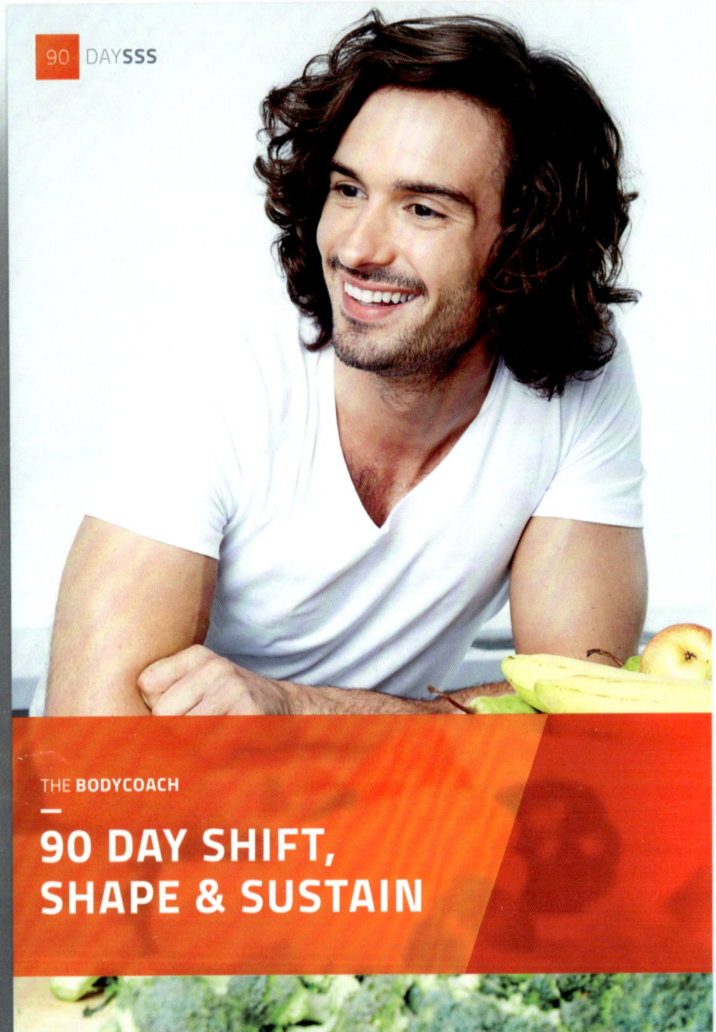
90 DAYSSS
THE BODYCOACH
90 DAY SHIFT, SHAPE & SUSTAIN